Dr. Ghada Bouslama

Deep fungal infections of the oral cavity

Dr. Ghada Bouslama

Deep fungal infections of the oral cavity

Clinical diagnosis and treatment

ScienciaScripts

Cover image: www.ingimage.com

This book is a translation from the original published under ISBN 978-620-6-72248-9.

Publisher:
Sciencia Scripts
is a trademark of
Dodo Books Indian Ocean Ltd. and OmniScriptum S.R.L publishing group

120 High Road, East Finchley, London, N2 9ED, United Kingdom
Str. Armeneasca 28/1, office 1, Chisinau MD-2012, Republic of Moldova, Europe
Printed at: see last page
ISBN: 978-620-8-19878-7

Contents

Preface..2
Chapter 1..3
Chapter 2..11
Chapter 3..20
Chapter 4..29
Chapter 5..37
Chapter 6..40
Chapter 7..44
Conclusion...55
References...56

Preface

The oral cavity is a gateway to the human body offering a unique ecological environment and a variety of surfaces for colonisation, ranging from hard dental surfaces to keratinised and non-keratinised epithelium that sloughs off. It is not surprising that the oral cavity is home to a complex and dynamic microbiota, as it offers a number of pre-existing conditions favourable to the growth and proliferation of the oral microbiome, such as warmth, nutrition and humidity. In addition to the bacterial flora, around 85 species of fungi colonise the oral cavity, of which "Candida" is the most common and the main species associated with oral mycoses. Other fungi, such as Aspergillus, Cryptococcus, Histoplasma, Mucor Rhizopus, Coccidioides etc., are also capable of causing oral infections. These micro-organisms live in a saprophytic state. A simple disturbance of the oral balance can cause common or invasive infections that are difficult to treat, hence the term opportunistic infections. Superficial mycoses such as chronic candidiasis are generally associated with oral genetics, pain, burning, parageusia and difficulty in eating. On the other hand, the clinical presentation of invasive infections is varied, difficult to recognise and characterised by the spread of pathogenic agents into deep areas of tissue, causing an aggressive clinical presentation such as ulceration and bone lysis.

The incidence of deep oral mycoses has risen considerably due to the increasing prevalence of immunosuppressive conditions including AIDS, neoplastic diseases, unstable diabetes, bone marrow transplants, immunosuppressive therapy and prolonged use of corticosteroids.

Because of its opportunistic nature, commensal flora tend to become pathogenic in immunocompromised patients, and fungal disease can be much more resistant and invasive. Treatment is more complex, requiring knowledge of the cause of the disease, and can be life-threatening. Given the changing causes of immunodepression and the increasing prevalence of co-morbidities, it is essential to be able to detect, treat and, preferably, prevent oral mycoses in their invasive form.

In several chapters, this book presents the different clinical and radiological manifestations and diagnostic methods of deep mycoses of the orofacial region, enabling the practitioner to make an earlier and more accurate diagnosis in order to avoid the often fatal complications of these infections in immunocompromised patients, and to institute appropriate treatment.

Chapter 1

Characteristics of deep fungal infections

1. Guest features

1.1. Immunosuppression

1.1.1. Immunodepression linked to general pathology

► Uncontrolled diabetes

Chronic increase in blood glucose levels due to impaired insulin production by the B cells of the pancreas or inefficient use of insulin by the body (insulin resistance).

Rare infectious diseases such as invasive mycoses, and their associated comorbidities, are more common in diabetic patients than in the general population because of the associated mechanisms that impair the host's immune defence. These include suppression of cytokine production, defects in phagocytosis, a reduced immune response mediated by T lymphocytes, altered neutrophil function, inhibition of opsonisation mediated by immunoglobulins and the inability to kill microbes (7).

Poorly balanced diabetes is closely linked to fungal infections, by mucorales, Candida and aspergillus respectively.

Elevated glucose levels in the cell promote adhesion and tissue invasion and reinforce Candida virulence factors, particularly the enzymatic activity of phospholipases, esterases and hemolysins, increasing the pathogenicity, susceptibility and resistance of invasive candidiasis.

Given the weakness of the defence barrier in diabetics, the production of these enzymes is more intense, the lesion is more extensive and the severity of mucosal invasion is likely to be greater (41).

► The human immunodeficiency virus HIV/AIDS

It is one of the main causes of death in regions where resources are limited, as it attacks the immune system. Infected subjects are likely to contract haematological diseases, cardiac pathologies, gastrointestinal disorders and serious infections of the respiratory tract, ocular structures and central nervous system, thus aggravating the patient's immunodepressive state. Five malignant tumours have been found to be largely viral: Burkitt's lymphoma, immunoblastic lymphoma, primary central nervous system lymphoma, invasive cervical cancer and Kaposi's sarcoma.

Treatment of AIDS is associated with an increase in the number and function of CD4+ cells, leading to a dysregulated immune response to pathogens known as the inflammatory immune reconstitution syndrome, observed in 10-32% of seropositive patients. This syndrome is frequently attributed to opportunistic fungal infections, by any pathogen that can lead to the development of invasive and treatment-resistant forms of the disease (11). Over 90% of seropositive patients develop oral candidiasis at some point during the course of the disease (72). This is one of the earliest diagnostic indicators of AIDS, often in its pseudomembranous or erythematous form, such as angular cheilitis (52).

The problem arises when non-albicans Candida are isolated, most commonly Candida tropicalis, C. krusei, C. glabrata and C. parapsilosis: strains that are resistant to azoles and therefore difficult to treat. Seropositive patients have higher rates of colonisation by C. non-albicans than healthy individuals, due to their compromised immune status. Invasive candidiasis may develop in a seropositive subject through evolution of the superficial form or because of the abundance of non-albicans strains (40).

Invasive aspergillosis is a rare but devastating infection in patients with advanced AIDS, with a severity rate of 85.7%. HIV infection is associated with a poor prognosis because the underlying immunosuppression is progressive and, in most cases, irreversible. (37)

► **Hematological disorders**

There are quite a few affecting the quantity and function of blood cells and mainly immune cells.

► **Aplastic anemia**

It is part of the spectrum of bone marrow and blood cell diseases. It is associated with pancytopenia (reduction in the three blood lines) and hypocellular bone marrow when other diseases such as myelofibrosis, myelodysplasia and leukaemia are excluded. (61)

Invasive fungal infection is fairly common and is the main cause of death in these patients. Prolonged neutropenia due to the disease itself or its treatment (hematopoietic stem cell transplantation and immunosuppressive therapy) is one of the main risk factors for the development of invasive mycoses, frequently caused by Aspergillus species, followed by Zygomycetes, Candida spp and Fusarium spp (76).

► **Myelodysplastic syndromes**

Clonal disorders of bone marrow stem cells, characterised by inefficient hematopoiesis leading to blood cytopenias. Resulting clinical manifestations include anaemia, haemorrhage, infection and a high risk of leukaemia. Neutropenia is probably the main predisposing factor for severe fungal infections, in association with other immune deficiencies including altered neutrophil function, B, T and NK cell deficiencies and complications related to iron overload due to red cell transfusions (74).

► **Blood cancers**

Leukaemias, myelomas and lymphomas frequently develop from the various blood cells. Malignant haemopathies are responsible for severe and prolonged neutropenia, increasing the incidence of opportunistic infections such as invasive mycoses, with a high mortality rate. Candida albicans and Aspergillus remain the main pathogens identified. (64)

Leukaemia: myeloid or lymphoid, depending on the cells of origin, invades the bone marrow with abnormal cells that accumulate and subsequently interfere with the function of normal cells (risk of anaemia, bleeding and infection). Myeloid leukaemia is defined by the production and excessive accumulation of an abnormal sub-type of white blood cells: the PNN. Lymphocytic leukaemia develops at the expense of T or B lymphocytes (34).

The incidence of serious invasive mycoses is currently increasing in patients with acute leukaemia (64). Invasive candidiasis, in particular, occurs at an advanced stage of leukaemia, threatening the patient's vital prognosis (34). There is a high risk of developing invasive aspergillosis in refractory leukaemia, with a higher death rate given the underlying neutropenic state or associated cytotoxic treatment (37).

Lymphoma: Hodgkin's or non-Hodgkin's lymphoma, depending on the presence or absence of Reed-Sternberg tumour cells. It is a cancer of the lymphatic system that corresponds to malignant neoplastic mutations of the lymphoid stem cells. Lymphomas are characterised by the excessive proliferation of altered lymphocytes (usually B or T) in lymphoid organs such as the lymph nodes, spleen and liver. These altered blood cells can develop throughout the body, leading to a generalised alteration in the host's immune response (78).

Multiple myeloma develops at the expense of a particular type of white blood cell, the plasma cell. Their main property is the production of immunoglobulins (antibodies capable of organising an immune response targeted against an antigen). A tumour plasma cell multiplies excessively, produces large quantities of a single type of immunoglobulin, the monoclonal peak, and leads to the deregulation of healthy plasma cells, restricting the synthesis of normal antibodies. It may even invade the bone marrow and reduce the production of other immune cells, thereby reducing immune effectiveness in the face of infection. Bone fragility resulting from the destruction of bone by tumour plasma cells is a specific symptom of multiple myeloma (22).

1.1.2. Immunodepression linked to ongoing treatment

► Targeted therapies/ Chemotherapy

Chemotherapy is based on the use of drugs that directly destroy cancer cells and prevent them from multiplying. It temporarily blocks the activity of the bone marrow (medullary aplasia), leading to a reduction in the production of blood cells and therefore a weakening of the immune system, of variable duration. Leukopenia of neutrophils (neutropenia) or lymphocytes (lymphopenia) leads to an alarming reduction in immune defences, resulting in increased susceptibility to opportunistic

infections. The use of targeted biological therapies to treat malignant haemopathies is currently increasing.
Deficiencies in innate and cell-mediated immunity associated with cytotoxic chemotherapies, targeted immunotherapies and long-term intravenous catheters, together with chemotherapy-related loss of mucosal integrity, significantly increase the risk of fungal infection. Invasive mycoses are a major cause of morbidity and mortality in patients receiving immunosuppressive therapy. Yeast infections, including invasive candidiasis, mould infections such as aspergillosis, endemic fungal diseases such as histoplasmosis or blastomycosis, and classic opportunistic infections such as cryptococcosis, are serious complications associated with antineoplastic treatments and have been progressively increasing in recent years. (38)
The presence of Candida tropicalis in mucosal surveillance cultures has been reported to be a poor predictor of subsequent invasive mycosis in neutropenic patients. Patients receiving high-dose myelosuppressive chemotherapy prior to stem cell transplantation currently benefit from systematic antifungal prophylaxis (33).

► **Organ or hematopoietic stem cell transplants**

Neutropenia is consecutive to conditioning, due to intensification of potent immunosuppressive therapy against graft versus host disease, graft rejection and cytomegalovirus disease (62).
Solid organ transplantation is associated with a high risk of fungal infections, mainly aspergillosis, generally during the first year of transplantation (62). The occurrence of aspergillosis and the highest rate of letalitis are observed respectively in liver transplants (67.6%), kidney transplants (62.5%), lung transplants and cniir transplants (37). Infections occur in approximately 5% of lung transplant recipients and are mainly caused by Candida and Aspergillus (62).

► **Hematopoietic stem cell transplant recipients** are at high risk of invasive aspergillosis because of the gross intensity of immunosuppression. Factors implicated include receipt of T-cell depleted or selected stem cell products, receipt of corticosteroids, neutropenia and lymphopenia (62).

► **Corticosteroids**

These drugs are commonly used and are characterised by their immunosuppressive and anti-inflammatory effects, exerted via glucocorticoid receptors that oppose the activity of the essential transcriptional regulators of leukocyte pro-inflammatory genes. The immune deficiency caused by corticotherapy is summarised in these phenomena:

- Reduce the number of monocytes and macrophages by inhibiting their myelopoiesis and release into the bone marrow.

- To inhibit phagocytic function during high-dose glucocorticoid therapy with an immediate risk of infection, particularly in hematopoietic stem cell transplant recipients and patients with autoimmune diseases such as disseminated lupus erythematosus.
- > A major risk factor in the development of chronic pulmonary aspergillosis, invasive aspergillosis, fungal keratitis and other invasive fungal infections. (36)

Corticosteroids have profound effects on the distribution and function of neutrophils, monocytes and lymphocytes. In addition, corticosteroids directly stimulate the growth of Aspergillus. In vitro, Aspergillus fumigatus presents sterol-binding proteins. (62)

Apart from their immunosuppressive effect, corticosteroids are responsible for disturbing the oral balance through their xerostomal side-effects and alteration of the interaction between the bacterial and fungal microbiome, thus creating an environment favourable to fungal colonisation and growth (47).

Boven and Vegter (13) carried out an analysis and found that after one year of treatment with corticosteroids, 701 patients had received medication for oral candidiasis, whereas one year before administration, only 361 patients had received antifungals, so an increased risk of oral candidiasis is linked to corticotherapy. The incidence of this infection over three years in patients on treatment was 7.3%. However, a higher dose increases the incidence of oral candidiasis, which reduces compliance with these drugs. (13)

- **Broad-spectrum antibiotics**

May also disrupt commensal microbial communities and affect host immune competence, increasing susceptibility to infection. Several immune alterations are associated with the administration of broad-spectrum antibiotics, such as a reduction in the number of CD8+ cells in the colon. The absence of intestinal microbial stimuli led to a decrease in cytokine production by CD4+ cells, a decrease in the percentage of memory/effector T cells, regulatory T cells and active dendritic cells in the grafted intestine, colon, spleen and mesenteric lymph nodes. This immune deficiency will therefore play an important role in the development of opportunistic infectious diseases. (24) Despite their underestimated incidence, invasive fungal infections are important emerging complications of late morbidity and mortality, especially in hospitalised patients. (69)

1.2. Development of resistance to antifungal agents

Compared with antibiotics, antifungal drugs are limited in number and mechanism of action. Effective treatment of invasive fungal infections is generally based on three main classes of antifungal agents: azoles, echinocandins and polyenes. The widespread use of these drugs has altered the epidemiology of infections, given the tendency of fungi to develop resistance, thereby limiting therapeutic options and often leading to treatment failure, especially if other factors such as toxicities or drug interactions come into play.

Drug resistance is mainly linked to the increase in the number of patients at increased risk of invasive fungal infection due to complex surgical procedures or immunodepression. The current emergence of fungi resistant to antifungal agents is very worrying, which is why we need to know the main mechanisms of resistance within the three classes of antifungal agents, as well as the clinical implications for the treatment of fungal infections. (2)

1.2.1. Resistance to azoles

Fluconazole, voriconazole and posaconazole are the most commonly prescribed. Azoles inhibit fungal growth by acting on the enzyme lanosterol 14a-demethylase, which is responsible for converting lanosterol into ergosterol (a key component of the fungal cytoplasmic membrane).

Resistance to azoles results from the expression of drug efflux pumps and mutations in the ERG11 gene which lead to a reduction in azole binding affinity (the ERG11 gene is normally responsible for excessive biosynthesis of ergosterol, the target of azoles). Candida, particularly non-albicans species, are capable of developing resistance to azoles. C. glabrata, C. tropicalis and C. krusei often display intrinsic resistance to fluconazole. In addition to the extracellular matrix of Candida, the ease with which it forms a biofilm housing high-density micro-organisms acts as a physical barrier to azole penetration.

Resistance in Aspergillus is mainly due to ABC transport proteins which reduce intracellular azole concentrations by efflux and to mutations in the cyp51A gene which codes for lanosterol 14a-demethylase. Excessive production of the enzyme is also possible, submerging the antifungal azole at therapeutic concentrations. (39)

- Azoles are widely used in the clinical, agricultural and industrial sectors, which explains the ability of Aspergillus to develop resistance to medicinal triazoles, requiring the use of other therapeutic molecules, such as liposomal amphotericin B, when the prevalence of azole resistance is high (i.e. > 10%). (4)

1.2.2. Resistance to echinocandins

The echinocandins (micafungin, caspofungin and anidulafungin), used intravenously, represent a very important class, particularly in the treatment of invasive candidiasis. Echinocandins act by inhibiting the synthesis of 1,3-e-D-glucan, an essential component of the fungal cell wall. This mechanism is different from that of azole antifungals, and it is for this reason that echinocandins have generally retained their activity against most azole-resistant Candida species. However, C. glabrata is able to develop resistance to echinocandins because :

- Mutations in the FKS1 gene of 1,3-e-D-glucan synthase, the most common origin, give rise to amino acid substitutions that significantly reduce affinity for echinocandins.

- Increased chitin production in response to reduced glucan synthesis is associated with reduced sensitivity to echinocandins (39).

1.2.3. Polyene resistance

Polyenes alter the permeability of the cell membrane by creating pores, binding to ergosterol and causing leakage of intracellular contents. Resistance to amphotericin B affects ergosterol synthesis through mutation of the ERG genes. It is rare to find species resistant to amphotericin B, as it is a broad-spectrum antifungal agent (administered parenterally, in its liposomal form). Amphotericin B remains the cornerstone of treatment for invasive mucosal infections, as well as an alternative therapy for severe infections with azole-resistant moulds. (39)

2. Fungal virulence factors

Fungi are eukaryotes that take the form of yeasts, moulds or dimorphs. Primary pathogenic fungi, once in the human body, proliferate almost exclusively in the form of yeast, from which they can easily spread to distant sites by passing into the bloodstream and extracellular fluid (31). Some fungi, if inhaled in large quantities, rarely cause invasive mycoses in immunocompetent individuals. If the immune system is compromised, commensal agents tend to become pathogens and their virulence factors are favoured, leading to systemic mycoses affecting the oral cavity and several organs and systems. (2)

2.1. Cell adhesion

Fungi are able to adhere to tissues and prevent their elimination by ciliary action or viscous membranes thanks to adhesion molecules such as Als, Hwplp, Cshlp... (2)

C. albicans, for example, is able to adhere to oral epithelial cells and form a biofilm, increasing its pathogenicity thanks to several adhesion molecules and multiple phenomena such as physical forces (van der Waals interactions), hydrophobicity and electrostatic bonding (68).

A. fumigatus is characterised by hydrophobic proteins, such as galactomannan and chitin, covering the conidia and facilitating adhesion to albumin and collagen (2).

2.2. Dimorphism

In other words, the ability to change from a commensal, non-pathogenic form to a pathogenic form that causes mycoses. Yeasts have round or ovoid cells, which divide by binary fission and produce a distinct, independent daughter cell. Moulds are filamentous and grow by apical extension. They produce hyphae or mycelium, which may be branched but united with the mould, enabling it to invade tissues. Some fungi may have additional morphotypes or transient forms such as pseudohyphae in C. albicans (2).

2.3. Thermotolerance

Ability to grow at high temperatures > 37°C. Most thermopathogenic fungi resemble moulds at room temperature and are able to evolve from one form to another at different temperatures. A. fumigatus develops at high T°s of up to 55°C. In C. albicans, the transition from one form to another depends on environmental changes linked to temperature and pH. (2)

2.4. Presence of a capsule

The presence of a polysaccharide capsule limits the functioning of the complement system, blocks the circulation of leukocytes in the infected area and deregulates the release of cytokines (2).

2.5. Enzyme and protein release

Pathogenic fungi are capable of releasing degradation enzymes responsible for tissue destruction and immune weakening, thus facilitating the spread of disease. Proteases and phospholipases are found in the majority of fungi, such as C.albicans, Aspergillus fumigatus, Cryptococcus neoformans and Coccidioides. Some enzymes are produced to neutralise the toxic oxygen released by neutrophils and macrophages.

Melanin production inhibits antibody-mediated phagocytosis. It protects the fungi against severe conditions such as high temperatures and UV rays (2).

2.6. Acquisition of iron

Iron is necessary for the development of fungi, but is generally bound to proteins in humans. Therefore, they call upon three iron absorption mechanisms such as absorption by Fe reductase, absorption of ferrous iron and absorption by siderophores (iron chelators synthesised by fungi). (2)

Chapter 2

Invasive oral candidiasis

1. Epidemiology

Oral candidiasis is an often superficial opportunistic infection that can occur in immunocompetent or immunodepressed patients. Its invasive form is rare, and more closely related to immunodepression (12). Invasive candidiasis is the most common of the invasive mycoses. It includes Candida bloodstream infections (candidemia) and deep tissue infections. Deep-tissue candidiasis results either from hematogenic dissemination or direct inoculation of candida species. It is a locally destructive infection, associated with high morbidity and mortality rates of up to 40%, and can lead to systemic infection (32).

According to conservative estimates (32), invasive candidiasis affects more than 250,000 people worldwide every year and is responsible for 50,000 deaths. Candidiasis is the 4eme most common blood infection. The diagnosis of invasive candidiasis should be made in patients presenting with neutropenia and unexplained fever that do not respond to antibiotics. (32)

The breakdown of the mucocutaneous barrier in the immunocompromised becomes a gateway for Candida and, after an episode of fungemia, Candida can localise in any deep tissue (5).

Pathogenesis is complex and influenced by colonisation, alteration of physical barriers and phagocytic responses - facilitating transformation into opportunism which introduces important virulence factors at the origin of infection. In an immunocompromised individual, superficial candidiasis can easily develop into a severe invasive form, accumulating in vital organs and causing disseminated candidiasis (12).

Invasive candidiasis manifests itself in the form of candidemia, disseminated infections, osteomyelitis, mucocutaneous infection and rhinosinusitis. Their clinical presentation may be unspecific, complicating diagnosis and delaying treatment, thereby jeopardising the patient's survival. In the absence of a rapid and accurate diagnosis, empirical treatment should be instituted (42).

2. Etiopathogeny

Candida is part of the normal oral microflora, as a commensal rather than pathological population. Approximately 30-60% of adults and 45-65% of infants carry Candida species in their oral cavities. (72)

Candida albicans are the most isolated **type** in over 80% of lesions.

Although C. albicans is the dominant pathogen, non-albicans species are increasingly encountered in the diagnosis of invasive candidiasis (42). These include :

Candida dublieniesis: morphologically and genotypically similar to C. albicans, often identified in HIV-infected patients. It forms true hyphae and is less sensitive to fluconazole.

Candida glabrata is characterised by its rapid growth and resistance to fluconazole, leading to more serious and difficult-to-treat deep blood and mucous membrane infections.

Candida krusei: common in people with HIV or hematological disorders due to the widespread use of fluconazole prophylaxis.

Candida tropicalis: secretes moderate levels of proteinases and adheres strongly to epithelial cells. This is the most virulent non-albicans species, with the greatest resistance to commonly used antifungal agents. It is generally isolated from the skin and oral cavity and is responsible for resophageal infections in patients suffering from systemic diseases.

Candida parapsilosis: mainly in critically ill newborns and patients in intensive care units because of its ability to adhere to medical devices and its tendency to colonise the skin (19).

The increased frequency of candidiasis in immunocompromised individuals is linked to a number of Candida spp virulence factors, such as the ability to adhere effectively to epithelial and endothelial cells, phenotypic change, yeast-hyphal transition, biofilm-forming ability, hydrophobicity and enzymatic activity. Candida species secrete extracellular enzymes that play an important role in pathogenesis, invasion, tissue destruction and the onset of clinical signs. Phospholipases and esterases are responsible for tissue invasion and hemolysins for lysing blood cells (41).

Candida species differ considerably in terms of virulence. C. albicans, C. tropicalis and C. glabrata are more virulent than C. krusei and C. parapsilosis, which are respectively very rare (32).

Candida are characterized by resistance to fluconazole and sometimes to echinocandins, either intrinsic, as in the case of fluconazole resistance in C. krusei, or acquired as a result of high use of the antifungal agent (44).

3. Systemic factors aggravating oral candidiasis

Invasive candidiasis is a progressive process evolving in several stages, from colonisation to invasive infection. In an immunocompetent patient, the healthy skin and mucous membranes defend themselves effectively against infection. The progressive expansion of colonisation, immunodepression and the breakdown of mucocutaneous barriers secondary to invasive therapies or a pathological process provide the breeding ground for Candida infections, which are true opportunistic infections. In addition to local risk factors, such as the wearing of ill-fitting dentures, smoking and alcohol consumption, local trauma caused by dental extraction or other surgery, and hyposalivation, other more important general factors must be taken into account. (72)

Generally, invasive candidiasis is an infection secondary to any state of immunodepression, mainly in patients with severely compromised defence mechanisms. These include HIV/AIDS, the use of steroids or broad-spectrum antibiotics, malignant tumours, chemotherapy, organ transplantation, bone marrow transplantation, intravenous drug users, multiple organ failure, poorly balanced diabetes, malnutrition, extreme age (newborns and the elderly), parental hyperalimentation, etc. (5)
In addition to the predisposing factors initially described, we add :

► **Dietary deficiencies**

The role of iron deficiency in the development of oral candidiasis has been demonstrated through at least four mechanisms which make the oral mucosa more susceptible to infection:

- Risk of epithelial abnormalities such as hyperkeratosis and atrophy due to alterations in the kinetics of rapidly dividing mucosal cells, which in turn result from alterations in iron-dependent enzyme systems.
- Depression of cell-mediated immunity both in vivo and in vitro.
- Defects in phagocytosis.
- Inadequate production of antibodies.

Thus, deficiencies in vitamins A, B1, B2, C, folic acid, magnesium and zinc are generally implicated in the occurrence of candidiasis. (68)

► **Other factors**

Their ability to multiply in several parenteral nutrition solutions can trigger candidiasis. Lipid solutions encourage germination and biofilm formation. Similarly, high serum glucose concentrations favour biofilm formation and pathogenicity.
Critically ill patients, for example those with renal failure, are at risk of invasive candidiasis due to immune dysfunction and renal replacement therapy via a vascular catheter. Patients with sepsis or septic shock have several factors favouring infection, such as invasive therapeutic strategies (implanted medical devices, source control surgery), intestinal barrier dysfunction and sepsis-induced immunosuppression (73).

4. Clinical and radiological forms and manifestations

Superficial candidiasis, in its pseudomembranous, erythematous, hyperplastic, angular cheilitis, dental stomatitis and median rhomboid glossitis forms, is easily diagnosed and treated by eliminating the local etiology responsible for the disturbance in oral balance. However, invasive forms of candidiasis are defined as locally aggressive or disseminated, requiring special diagnostic and therapeutic methods. A variety of clinical manifestations are observed in immunocompromised patients, ranging from mucosal destruction (ulcerations, necrotic plaques) to bone destruction and dissemination.

4.1. Candidiasis osteomyelitis

A fairly rare manifestation of invasive candidiasis. It is an inflammatory state of the bone and bone marrow resulting from a chronic, progressive infection starting in the medullary cavity, rapidly involving the haversian system and spreading to the periosteum of the region. The bones most frequently affected are the spine, femur, ribs, sternum and humerus. Candidiasis osteomyelitis is very rarely seen in the maxillofacial region. The high vascularity, porous nature and thin cortices of the maxilla compared to the mandible make it a less favoured site of infection. The mandible is the bone most frequently affected in the head and neck region.

Osteomyelitis is most often bacterial in origin. Fungal osteomyelitis is much less common and much more debilitating. Candida osteomyelitis can lead to significant bone destruction and high morbidity, particularly when its diagnosis and treatment are delayed because Candida spp is not recognised as a potential bone pathogen. (30)

Hematogenous dissemination is the most common mechanism of infection, followed by direct inoculation and infection by contiguity. Symptoms are localised in most cases, insidious in onset and sulbugue to chronic in course, with a moderate or minimal inflammatory response, so the most common symptom is local pain. (26)

This inflammatory process leads to compression of the blood vessels, resulting in bone necrosis. The aggressiveness of the infection can be devastating, as with mucormycosis, it can affect the maxillary alveolar process as well as the basal bone, part of the nasal bone in the course of the aigneous evolution and the sinus walls by contiguity. A necrotizing ulceration on the hard palate subsequently develops into a progressive perforation with nasal regurgitation of food and halitosis (30). The exposed bone is brown, dark yellowish in colour. The buccal vestibule is partially obliterated by diffuse rubbery soft tissue (6). In advanced stages, new signs may appear, such as yellowish crusts all around, nauseating discharge and a large septal perforation leading to saddle nose deformity (30). Involvement of the maxillary sinus with a complaint of sinusitis is a specific feature of the disease. (75)

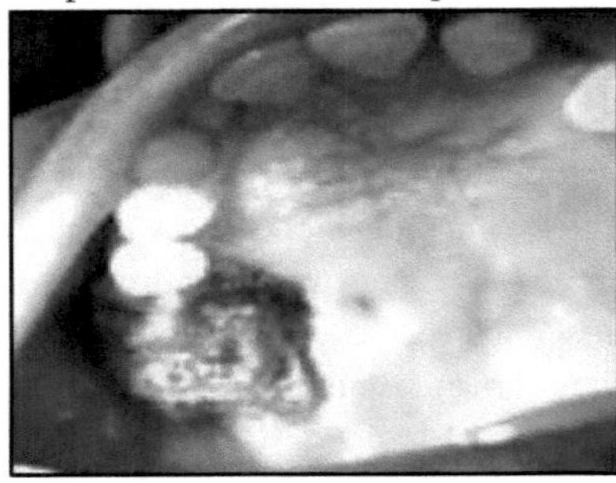

Figure 1: Intraoral view of necrotic bone exposed following Candida infection (65)

Panoramic radiography and tomodensitometry reveal the rupture of bony cortices, irregular lytic destruction of alveolar processes and nasal and/or sinus walls... with an impression of sequestration formation. The radiological features of osteolysis are more evident in young patients, particularly in mandibular lesions. (65)

4.2. Invasive candidiasis rhinosinusitis

It is a potentially fatal infection frequently associated with an altered neutrophil response. Invasive sinonasal candidiasis is as rare as it has not been widely described. It is currently discovered as a sequel to COVID-19 infection. The most common strains are C. parapsilosis, C. albicans, C. tropicalis and sometimes mixed infections.

Clinically, invasive sinonasal candidiasis presents as complicated sinusitis, with atypical symptoms including nasal involvement (crusts, nasal obstruction, facial pain), orbital involvement (ptosis, chemosis, proptosis, "deme, ophthalmoplegia), neurological involvement and intracranial extension.

Of the 475 cases of fungal rhinosinusitis, 18 had candidal infection involving the nose and sinuses, two had orbital involvement without loss of vision, 3 had intracranial extension and 1 had pulmonary involvement. The mandible was involved in only one patient, while the maxilla and palate were involved in five patients (8). Isolated nasal infection is extremely rare. It is usually associated with primary maxillary osteomyelitis. (30)

Non-contrast computed tomography of the paranasal sinuses is generally the first test of choice, while MRI is used if extra-sinus extension to the soft tissues is suspected. (8)

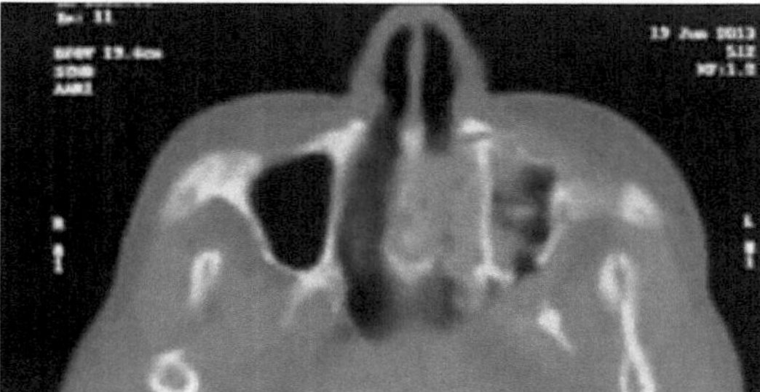

Figure 2: CT axial section showing bone lysis on the left maxillary side, sinus filling and invasion of the nasal cavity (65).

4.3. Deep mucocutaneous candidiasis

(This is the form identified in our 1er clinical case). Primary deep cutaneous-mucosal candidiasis is a rare form of invasive candidiasis in which candida is present in deep cutaneous structures but has not yet disseminated. It is characterised by a variety of morphologies, ranging from papules or papulopustular plaques to necrotic plaques, enabling superficial candidiasis to be distinguished from deep candidiasis. The invasive form generally takes the form of disseminated acneiform necrotic papules associated with myalgia and fever. The clinical presentation is more suggestive of mucormycosis and differs from the appearance of superficial infections (white patches). The differential diagnosis includes invasive fungal infection, neutrophilic dermatosis, leukaemia, lymphoma or melanoma (16).

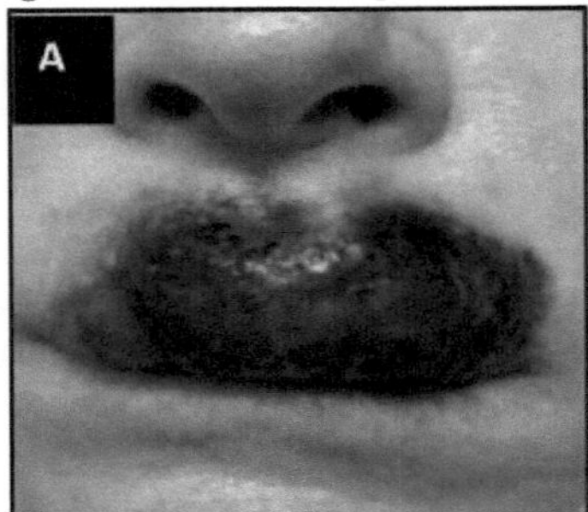

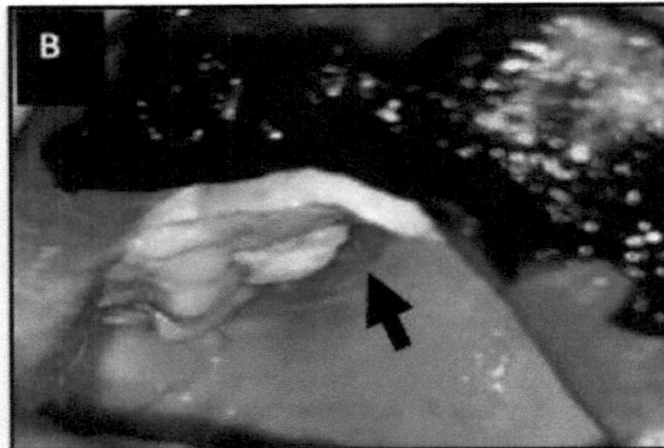

Figure 3. Clinical presentation of deep mucocutaneous candidiasis of the upper yeast (16)
A and B: purpuric ulcerous plaque affecting the upper yeast.
B: ulcerated, angular plaque with a violaceous border at the level of the hard palate on the right side and an upper labial ulceration which bleeds spontaneously.

4.4. The candidacy

The most common hematogenic fungal infection, since Candida are commensal inhabitants of the oropharynx and gastrointestinal tract. In addition to the initial risk factors for invasive candidiasis, candidemia is strongly associated with complicated immunodepressive states such as patients in intensive care units, hemodialysis, multiple blood transfusions, prolonged mechanical ventilation, gastrointestinal surgery and pancreatitis (23).

Oropharyngeal candidiasis is the most common and recurrent superficial infection in patients with AIDS or undergoing chemotherapy, and may progress to resophageal candidiasis or Candida resophagitis (46).

In critically ill patients, a possible correlation has been demonstrated between the pre-existence of oropharyngeal or resophageal candidiasis and the development of candidemia. Conversely, oropharyngeal/resophageal candidiasis is considerably more frequent in immunocompromised patients with previous candidemia (23).

5. Diagnostic tools

Although superficial candidiasis is easily recognised by its clinical aspects, the manifestations of deep candidiasis can be shaky by grouping together other invasive mycoses and neoplasms. The histological features of candidiasis are common to all fungal infections: mycotic infiltration of the blood vessels, vasculitis with thrombosis, infarction, haemorrhage and linear neutrophilic infiltration. As there are no specific clinical signs, clinicians rely on microbiological techniques to confirm the diagnosis, identify the species of Candida involved and control the disease in order to prevent the infection spreading further.

Biopsies are always necessary to rule out epithelial dysplasia or malignant transformation. A combination of the different diagnostic options provides an earlier and more sensitive diagnosis.

5.1. Histopathological examination

For candidal hyphae to be adequately visualised, biopsy tissues should be stained with specific stains such as Schiff's periodic acid (PAS), hematoxylin-eosin (H&E) or Grocott-Gomori methenamine silver (GMS). (68)

Histopathology shows pseudoseptate hyphae in clusters with budding yeast cells in focal areas. (6)

Direct microscopic examination of the biopsy tissues after the addition of a few drops of KOH can also give an idea of the nature of the infection (candidiasis) but not of the species of Candida involved. It is inconclusive, hence the need for a culture to help choose the right antifungal treatment.

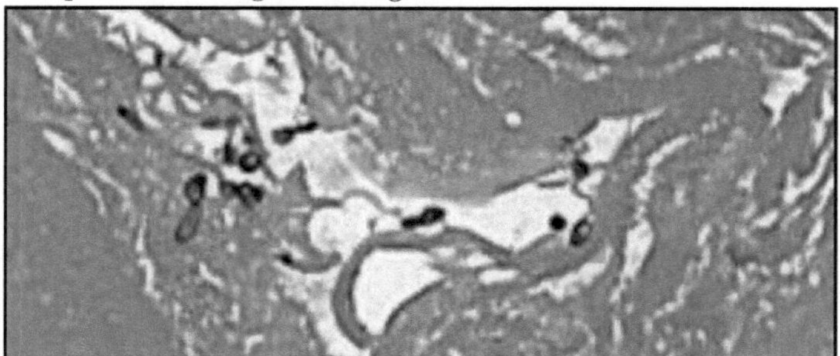

Figure 4: PAS stain showing budding yeasts with pseudohyphae suggestive of Candida species (16)

5.2. Cultivation

This is an essential diagnostic step, enabling the species or species involved to be detected, with a view to selecting the appropriate antifungal agent and avoiding resistance to treatment and hence recurrence of the infection. Culture dishes are used for macroscopic observation of Candida, with the addition of chloramphenicol 0.05 g/l or gentamycin 0.5 g/l to inhibit bacterial growth. The culture medium used is often Sabouraud dextrose gelose, which allows selective growth of the fungi. After incubation (24-48 hours), whitish cottony colonies are observed (15).

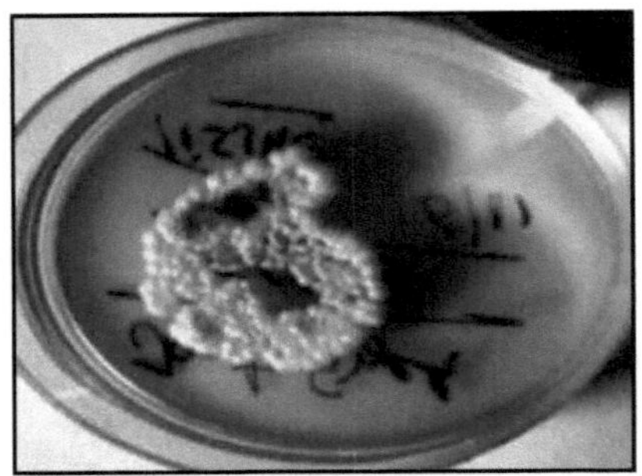

Figure 5. Culture plate showing the growth of Candida albicans (6)

5.3. Genetic techniques

The PCR test (SeptiFast and T2Candida Panel multiplex) (32) corresponds to nucleic acid hybridization and amplification techniques. The use of tests based on the polymerase chain reaction is effective for the detection of Candida, enabling the pathogenic agent to be identified without the need for cultures, while saving time and offering high sensitivity and specificity. These tests are still expensive (15). The PCR test has a sensitivity of 89% for deep candidiasis.

5.4. Immunological techniques: detection of antigens and antibodies

Are used in complicated clinical conditions when it proves difficult to obtain deep samples or when there are long waiting intervals between cultures (15). Mannans, antimannans and B-d-glucan are the main candidal markers.

B-D-glucan is a constituent of the fungal cell wall. The sensitivity of the test for Candida (Fungitec G) is generally high (76.7-100%).

Detection of mannans and antimannans (Candida Detect™) is also useful in establishing the diagnosis. (44)

6. Therapeutic management

The treatment of invasive candidiasis is based on three fundamental principles:

- Correcting predisposing factors and monitoring underlying diseases.
- The use of the most appropriate antifungal medicines.
- Surgical debridement of necrotic tissue.

6.1. Treatment with antifungal drugs

Antifungal treatment may be topical or systemic. Systemic antifungals are prescribed in cases of flagrant immunodepression to treat an infection which is widespread and/or invasive, due to its significant tissue destruction. (50) Nystatin is limited to the treatment of superficial candidiasis.

Fluconazole (Diflucan) 400 mg (6 mg/kg) per day remains the standard initial treatment for deep candidiasis and candidemia. The other triazoles have a broader spectrum of activity, but more limited indications for treatment. The duration of treatment should be adapted to the immune status, severity of infection and clinical response. The dosage of fluconazole and itraconazole (Sporanox) should be adjusted in cases of renal failure. The dosage of voriconazole (Vfend) should be adjusted in the presence of hepatic insufficiency.

-> High serum levels are often associated with the use of high doses or drug interactions, so liver function should be assessed at the start of treatment, every month, for the first three months and then periodically.

Initial treatment should be followed by prolonged antifungal treatment with fluconazole for 6 to 12 months (58).

Liposomal amphotericin B (3 to 5 mg/kg/day) becomes the treatment of choice in cases of intolerance to azoles, refractory infection or a virulent micro-organism (C.krusei ++). It is the 1st-line treatment in cases of bone involvement (osteomyelitis and invasive rhinosinusitis). (45)

Echinocandins IV are preferred in the event of detection of a fluconazole-resistant species or isolation of C. glabrata. (44)

Antifungal prophylaxis :

Other management options (prophylactic, preemptive and empirical) are used, as mortality is high in high-risk patients, to prevent the occurrence of invasive mycosis. Fluconazole is routinely administered, and recently echinocandins (45).

6.2. Surgical treatment

Antifungal treatment and timely surgery (debridement, curettage, sequestrectomy) lead to successful resolution of the disease. Regular clinical, radiological and laboratory follow-up for 2 years or more is necessary to prevent recurrence of the infection. (75)

Chapter 3

Orofacial mucormycosis

1. Epidemiology

Mucormycosis, zygomycosis or phycomycosis, is an invasive, opportunistic, rare but highly aggressive fungal infection. The disease is harmless in healthy individuals but fatal in immunocompromised patients, with diabetic ketoacidosis and neutropenia being common predisposing conditions. This infection has a remarkable affinity for the arteries. It is a potentially fatal infection with high morbidity and mortality. The fungus often alters the internal elastic lamina of the blood vessel media, damaging the endothelium and leading to thrombosis and therefore even widespread tissue necrosis of the oral and maxillofacial tissues. (35)
In the mouth, mucormycosis is the second most common fungal infection in humans after candidiasis. Although mucormycosis has been reported worldwide, it is more common in tropical and subtropical countries. The prevalence of mucormycosis is highest in India (14 cases/100,000 population), whereas it varies between 0.01 and 0.2 cases per 100,000 population in Europe and the United States. Mucormycosis is classified into five types according to the site and incidence of onset, with the rhino-orbito-cerebral form (34%) being the most widespread, followed by the cutaneous (22%), pulmonary (20%) and disseminated (13%) forms, gastrointestinal (8%) and in other unusual sites (3%) including the kidneys, middle ear, parotid gland, cuur, uterus, bladder, cervical lymph nodes and oral cavity.
The annual prevalence of mucormycosis is around 910,000 cases worldwide. If we exclude Indian data, there are only 10,000 cases worldwide per year. (35)

2. Etiopathology: Micro-organisms involved

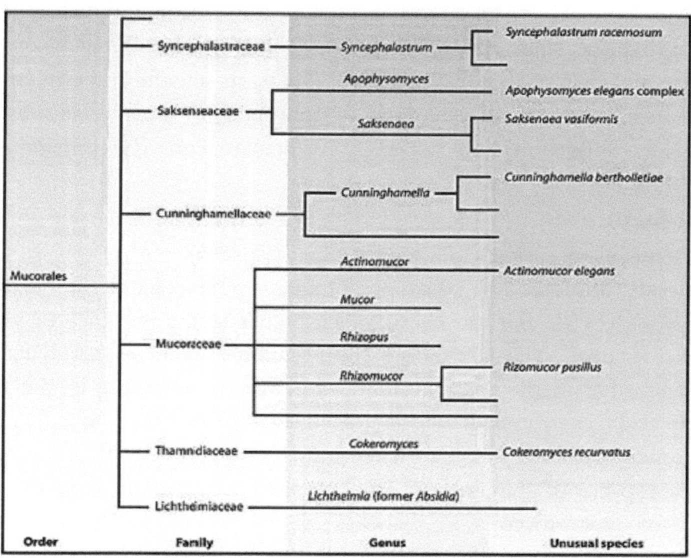

Figure 6. Species diversity of mucorales (28)

Mucormycosis is mainly caused by the family Mucoraceae, order Mucorales. The Mucor and Rhizopus species are the main causative agents. These micro-organisms are filamentous, ferrophilic, saprophytic and ubiquitous in nature, generally present in soil, animal excrement, agricultural debris or other organic matter. They develop rapidly in a moist environment, spread in the form of airborne propagules and are transmitted by three different routes, namely inhalation, ingestion and direct inoculation into an open wound. This infection is angioinvasive, since mucorales are characterised by their great affinity for the arteries. Cetone reductase, an enzyme secreted by mucorales, favours their development in hyperglycemic and acidic environments (diabetic acidocetosis +++). The siderophores of mucorales increase the absorption of iron, a necessary element for their growth and diffusion, thus encouraging tissue invasion. (71)

3. Disease site and pathophysiology

Oral mucormycosis is part of the rhino-orbito-cerebral form, which is the most widespread, accounting for around 1/3-1/2 of all cases, of which around 90% are affected by "Rhizopus". The maxillae and the four pairs of sinuses (frontal, sphenoidal, ethmoidal and maxillary) form an ideal niche, where the stable habitat of constant temperature and humidity allows these fungi to grow. Mucormycosis often starts in the nose and paranasal sinuses or in the palate and spreads rapidly to the air cavities and adjacent intracranial structures due to the diversity of communications at the base of the skull.

Early stage maxillofacial mucormycosis manifests as maxillary sinusitis and osteomyelitis mimicking pain or toothache. Clinical presentation includes potential early sinus drainage, sinus pressure, soft tissue tumefaction and may be increasingly progressive and diffuse to adjacent tissues due to its angioinvasive nature. In the advanced stage, mucormycosis may lead to thrombosis of the internal carotid artery with cerebral infarction and progress to hematogenic dissemination of the infection. (35)

4. Risk factors

Mucormycosis mainly affects immunodeprimes (95.45%).

Unbalanced diabetes is the predominant risk factor in maxillofacial mucormycosis (71%), and the risk is much higher in the presence of underlying diabetic ketoacidosis. This is a serious complication of diabetes, involving elevated blood acidity due to the toxic accumulation of ketone bodies in the blood. It favours an acidic environment with increased levels of free ferric ions favourable to fungal growth. Acidosis prevents chemotaxis of polynuclears and reduces the phagocytic capacity of granulocytes, affecting the host's immune capacity. The high incidence of mucormycosis in diabetics is also linked to the production of cetoreductase, which enables cetonic bodies to be used and survive in an acid environment (35).

Diabetes is the most common risk factor in the Middle East and North Africa region, followed by the use of corticosteroids, solid organ transplants, hematological malignancies and prolonged neutropenia. However, in Europe, hematological conditions are the most common underlying condition (50%), followed by diabetes (23%) and trauma (18%). This difference is due to other regional factors that influence the pathogenesis of mucormycosis, such as meteorological conditions (humidity, tropical and subtropical climates and high temperatures). The growth of mucorales and the concentration of airborne particles depend on seasonal changes in temperature and humidity. In the Middle East, airborne spore concentrations are higher in autumn than in summer, leading to an increase in the incidence of mucormycosis (18).

Nevertheless, mucormycosis can affect healthy individuals due to the role of local risk factors in the pathogenesis of this disease. For example, oral surgical trauma can damage local vascularisation, providing an entry point for microbes. Only 5.68% (5/88) of patients in good general condition develop mucormycosis secondary to dental extraction. Immune deficiency remains the main predisposing factor, creating an iron-rich environment, low pH, hyperglycemia and hyperosmolarity, all of which favour the growth of fungi (35).

Covid-19-mucormycosis co-infection: the mucormycosis-covid-19 association is becoming a matter of concern given the sudden increase in cases of mucormycosis/black fungus worldwide during the pandemic. In severe cases of COVID-19, a variety of sequelae are detected causing immunodepression and an environment favourable to fungal growth and development, thus increasing susceptibility to mucormycosis: ^The endothelial lesions, low pH, hyperglycemia and high iron levels associated with COVID favour angioinvasion and adhesion of mucorales.

The dramatic reduction in the total number of T cells, including the CD4+ and CD8+ groups in severe cases of covid-19.

^ Cytokine storms caused by increased inflammatory markers increase ferritin levels and reduce iron export ^ Iron overload in cells causes tissue damage and necrotic tissue -> cell death and release of iron into the circulation.

^The diabetogenic effect of COVID-19: ability to exacerbate pre-existing diabetes and precipitate diabetic acidocetosis, key risk factors for mucormycosis.

Corticotherapy is the mainstay of current treatment for severe COVID-19. In addition to their hyperglycemic effect, their increased use eliminates the phagocytic capacity of white blood cells, predisposing patients to fungal infections. Other drugs such as immunomodulators (tocilizumab) can increase susceptibility to mucormycosis co-infection.

Co-infection with a third micro-organism has also been reported, mainly aspergillosis. Among the systemic diseases associated with co-infected patients, diabetes is the most common. Hypertension is also present in 34.3% of patients. (63)

5. Clinical aspects

5.1. Extra-oral signs

Early symptoms of rhinocerebral mucormycosis usually include headache, fever, lethargy, sinus pain, sinusitis, mouth and/or facial pain, congestion, blood-tinged nasal discharge, ear symptoms, hyposmia or anosmia.

If it spreads to the orbit and/or periorbital region, it causes pre-septal and orbital cellulitis, periorbital dementia, proptosis, chemosis (conjunctival dementia), ophthalmoplegia (limited movement of the eyeball) and visual disturbance or loss. Involvement of the contralateral eye suggests invasion of the cavernous sinus and thrombosis (20).

5.2. Intra-oral signs

Mucosa-lined, air-filled sinuses encourage invasion of the oral cavity, resulting in purulent discharge, halitosis, gingival enlargement at the necks of the teeth, sudden tooth mobility, erosions of the alveolar bone, painful necrotic ulcerations and necrosis of the hard palate. The suggestive lesions are initially red, then violaceous and finally black when the tissues concerned undergo necrosis as a result of thrombosis of the blood vessels. Exposure of a black denuded bone is suggestive of mucormycosis, sometimes with the presence of a palatal fistula. Necrotic bedsores are a sign of rapid progression of the infection. (20)

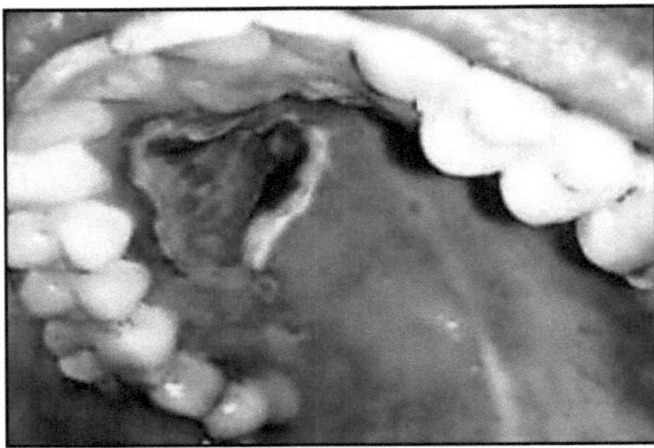

Figure 7. Clinical appearance of mucormycosis: mucosal ulceration and bone necrosis (49)

6. Radiological diagnosis

Preoperative **computed tomography (CT)** offers the best visualisation of the extent of the disease, thanks to axial and coronal sections and the injection of contrast medium. Maxillofacial mucormycosis usually manifests as maxillary sinusitis or multiple sinus involvement, which is often unilateral but can rapidly become bilateral. The CT scan shows thickening of the sinus mucosa or total filling of the sinuses, with confinement of the middle nasal cavity and destruction of the periorbital tissues and bone margins.

Embolisation of the maxillary, facial or ophthalmic arteries results in massive necrotic areas. CT angiography can be considered a necessary imaging modality for mucormycosis. Although sinus CT is the preferred imaging modality, the clinical course of mucormycosis usually precedes its radiological signs. (35)

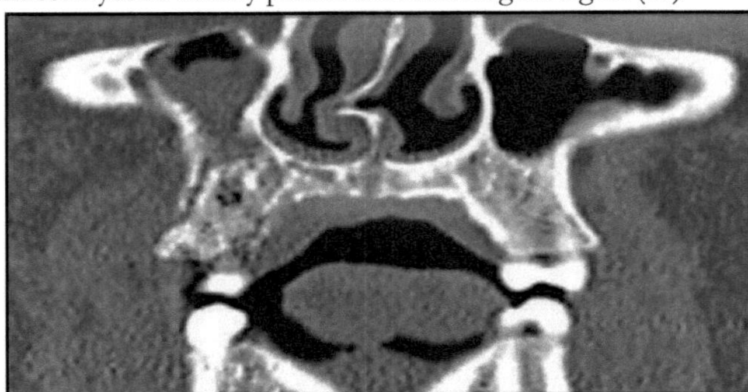

Figure 8. CT scan (frontal section): bone lysis and invasion of the maxillary sinus and nasal cavity on the right side (20).

Magnetic resonance imaging (MRI) is more sensitive than CT for exploring soft tissue involvement. It is useful for identifying extra-oral extensions (orbital, sinus, intradural, intracranial, etc.), thrombosis of the cavernous sinus, thrombosis of the cavernous portion of the internal carotid artery and perineural spread using contrast-enhanced MRI (56).

7. Diagnostic tools

Diagnosis of mucormycosis remains a formidable challenge for maxillofacial clinicians, given its rarity and the difficulty of obtaining deep tissue samples. Early, accurate and rapid diagnosis is essential to identify the pathogen, its antifungal susceptibility profile and to establish an effective treatment plan. Tissue biopsy is necessary.

7.1. Conventional methods

► Direct microscopic examination

Direct examination with the addition of potassium hydroxide (KOH), the use of fluorochromes or silver stains (GMS) can increase sensitivity in cases of low fungal density (27).

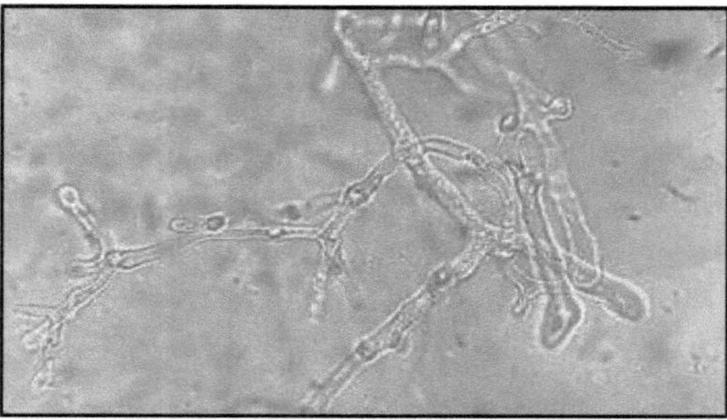

Figure 9. Direct microscopic examination showing large, sparsely septate fungal hyphae suggestive of mucormycosis (70).

► Mycological examination

Mucorales develop in 3 to 5 days at 25-30°C in most culture media, such as Sabouraud's gelose. (18)

► Histological diagnosis

This is the gold standard for diagnosing mucormycosis. Staining with hematoxylin and eosin (H&E), Grocott-Gomori methenamine-silver (GMS) or Schiff's periodic acid (PAS) reveals characteristically large (5-20 pm or more), thin-walled, ribboned, irregularly shaped, non-septate hyphae with branching at a wide angle (approximately 90°).

Histopathology also indicates a predominantly neutrophilic inflammatory response with large infarcts and angioinvasion. (35)

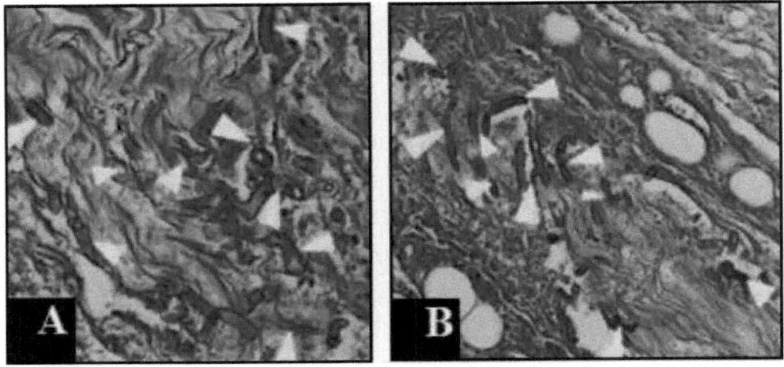

Figure 10: Histopathological examination of mucormycosis
A and B: Sinus tissue (400X magnification, PAS): Hyphae not septate, large and branched (35)

7.2. Diagnostic tools used more recently

Since their cell walls do not contain galactomannan or a significant amount of 1,3-b-D-glucan (BDG), neither the BDG test nor the galactomannan test is used to detect mucorales. (35)

DNA-based detection methods involve the amplification of genomic information via the chain polymerisation reaction. They are characterised by the use of mucosal-specific primers. (18) ► **Future prospects**

Technical developments and improvements are needed in the field of diagnostics, such as the use of a monoclonal antibody (2DA6) that reacts strongly with the fucomannan in Mucor.

A lateral flow test enables rapid and accurate detection of Rhizopus delemar, Lichtheimia corymbifera, Mucor circinelloides and Cunninghamella bertholletiae.

Another diagnostic approach is the evaluation of CD154+ T cells, which are considered new biomarkers since they are more numerous in patients with mucormycosis (18).

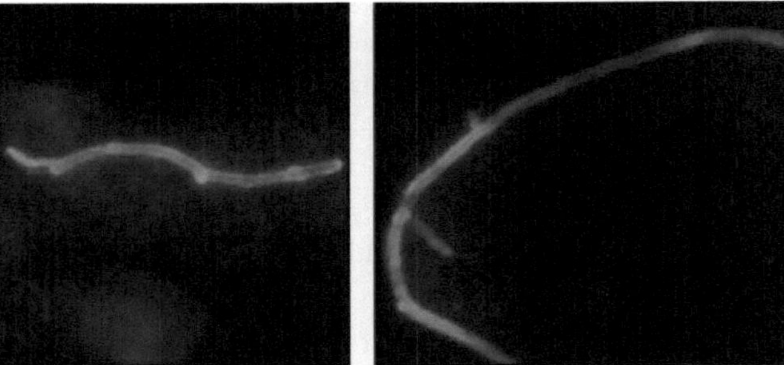
Figure 11. Branching angles of fluorescently stained mucorales. (35)

8. Treatment

Keys to successful therapy include suspicion of diagnosis with early recognition of clinical and radiological signs, correction of underlying medical conditions and aggressive medical and surgical intervention. Prophylactic oral administration of posaconazole can be used in neutropenic patients or patients with graft-versus-host disease (35).

8.1. Surgical debridement

Radical debridement with infection-free margins is performed as soon as possible to increase the patient's chances of recovery and survival, and to limit the fulminant spread of infection to adjacent structures.

Identification of surgical margins can be performed in real time using a fluorescent agent on infected tissue to avoid unnecessary resection of healthy tissue in craniofacial areas.

Sometimes, total resection of the maxillary arch or complete removal of the infected sinuses is necessary, along with aggressive debridement of the retro-orbital space (adipose tissue) to prevent the necrotic infection spreading into the millet.

Complete debridement, including endoscopic debridement and excision of infected tissue, increases survival rates. Regular follow-up after the operation is essential to detect new necrosis early, which must be treated by repeated debridement.

The defect resulting from debridement is often extensive, necessitating subsequent reconstructive surgery with a pedicle flap rather than a free flap, given the fungal affinity for blood vessels and the poor blood circulation of free flaps. An obturator prosthesis of the buccosinusal communication should be performed (35).

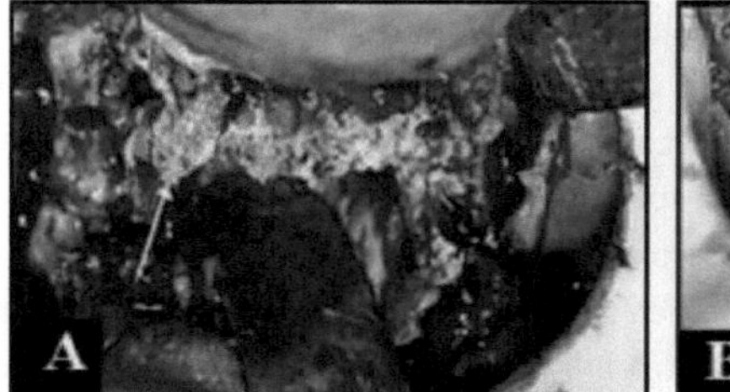

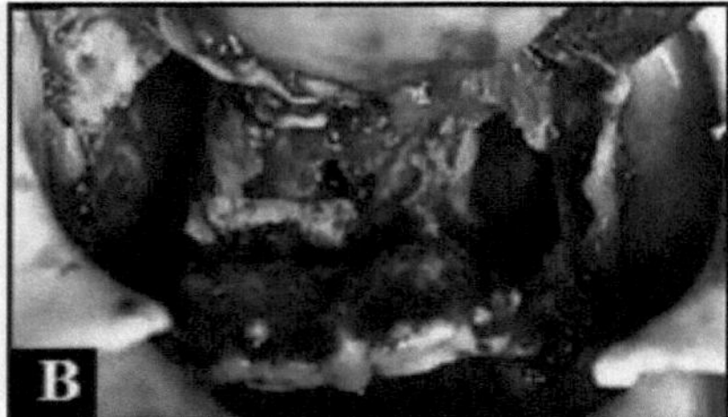

Figure 12. A: maxillary bone necrosis a cureter. B: appearance after debridement extended surgical (70)

8.2. Antifungal treatment

Early initiation of antifungal therapy at the first signs of mucormycosis can reduce the mortality rate to some extent.

Amphotericin B (AMB), whether conventional or liposomal, is probably the basic treatment to be applied with success. AMB deoxycholate at the highest tolerable dose (1.0-1.5 mg/kg/d) administered IV has been widely used. Its use is limited by frequent side-effects, mainly dose-limiting nephrotoxicity. Most of the negative side effects can be avoided by using lipid preparations of amphotericin B (LAMB). Liposomal AMB (5-10 mg/kg/d) has become the empirical drug of choice against Mucor species. (35)

This lipid-based formulation increases circulation time and modifies the biodistribution of the associated AMB. Complex drugs with lipid vehicles remain in the vascular system for longer. They may localise in higher concentrations in infected tissues (which have greater capillary permeability to lipid forms than healthy tissues). At the infected site, the drug is released by the action of lipases from the surrounding inflammatory cells. Liposomal AMB is less nephrotoxic than the conventional form. However, there are concerns about its dose-dependent hepatotoxicity (56).

Posaconazole (800 mg/d divided into 4 doses) is the 2[eme] drug of choice for mucormycosis, with minimal side effects. (35)

Isavuconazole (200 mg 3 times a day for 2 days and 200 mg a day thereafter) is the 3[eme] intention antifungal treatment. It can be administered orally or intravenously. It is less hepatotoxic than other azoles and is better tolerated than liposomal amphotericin B. It is often used as a complementary oral therapy after initial treatment with AMB. (20) Systemic treatment with high-dose liposomal amphotericin B is strongly recommended, while intravenous isavuconazole and intravenous posaconazole are recommended with moderate strength. Despite its nephrotoxicity, AMB desoxycholate is sometimes the only possible therapeutic option. (35)

8.3. Hyperbaric oxygen therapy

An effective complement to the current therapeutic approach involving exposure to 100% oxygen for 90 minutes to 2 hours under a pressure of 2 to 2.5 atm, one or 2 exposures per day for a total of 40 treatments. In addition to its fungicidal effect, it reduces acidosis and promotes neovascularisation and subsequent healing in poorly irrigated but viable acidotic and hypoxic tissues. (56)

Even after aggressive and appropriate medical and surgical treatment, the prognosis for mucormycosis remains poor, with a mortality rate varying between 25% and 80%, depending on the extent of the disease, the underlying risk factors and the rapidity of treatment. (43). Therefore, early diagnosis by an ENT or dental physician significantly improves the prognosis.

Chapter 4

Aspergillosis

1. Epidemiology

Aspergillosis is a rare fungal infection, invasive in immunocompromised individuals, caused by the Aspergillus species. It is a filamentous fungus and only a few strains are pathogenic for humans. Aspergillosis is a common infection of the respiratory tract, including the paranasal sinuses and oral cavity, with the possibility of life-threatening complications. (17)

Non-invasive infections resident in allergic sinusitis and aspergilloma, causing destruction of the sinus mucosa and bone atrophy.

Invasive aspergillosis of the paranasal sinuses is divided into limited (chronic or indolent) or fulminant (acute) invasive disease, with a rapid course progressing to destruction of the sinuses, nasal cavity, oral cavity and adjacent structures such as the orbit and brain within a few days.

Sinonasal aspergillosis is rarely reported in immunocompetent patients. It remains an invasive opportunistic infection that spreads through tissue layers. (48)

Oral aspergillosis is fairly rare and usually appears on the palate or tongue as a painful necrotic lesion. Once Aspergillus has inoculated the oral epithelium, its hyphae can penetrate tissues releasing toxins and can also disseminate hematogenously, causing secondary thrombosis and haemorrhage leading to tissue necrosis and rapid systemic infection. (17)

2. Etiopathology

Aspergillus infections have become increasingly important in recent years, due to the diversity and difficulty of accurately identifying the species. Aspergillus is ubiquitous in nature, in saprophytic form in air, water, soil, nutrients and decomposing organic matter. It has long been exploited as a biotechnological source for the production of pharmaceuticals, food ingredients and enzymes, and for the fermentation of soya, rice, cereals and potatoes. Aspergillus fumigatus is the main pathogen, followed by Aspergillus flavus.

The Fumigati section of Aspergillus comprises 63 species. These are heat-tolerant species, as they are capable of growing at high temperatures of up to 50°C. In addition to the Fumigati, a wide variety of sections are clinically relevant, including the species-rich Flavi, Nidulantes, Nigri, Terrei and Usti sections (4).

Among the many virulence factors present in Aspergillus are :

- The cell wall, with its dynamic structural properties and its protective role against external aggression.
- Its plasticity in the acquisition and metabolism of nutrients in the case of insufficient nutrient supply, necessary for fungal growth.

- Their ability to survive and develop in low oxygen conditions.
- The ability of the respiratory epithelium to escape fungal clearance: the first line of defence against inhaled conidia (4).
- The production of mycotoxins potentially harmful to human beings

A. Flavus is the main aflatoxin-secreting complex (29).

- The ability to cause co-infection with viruses, including the cytomegalovirus, the influenza virus, which leads to complications in the management of affected patients. (4)

3. Predisposing factors

The increased incidence of invasive aspergillosis is strongly associated with severe and/or prolonged neutropenia. The profile of patients at risk of invasive aspergillosis continues to expand, due respectively to malignant haemopathies and the use of intensive and aggressive cytotoxic treatments (in the treatment of malignant tumours and hematopoietic stem cell or solid organ transplants). Despite the progress made in current treatments, invasive aspergillosis remains a devastating opportunistic infection in immunocompromised patients, with an overall mortality rate of 58%. (37)

4. Characteristic clinical manifestations and pathogenesis

4.1. Pathogenesis

The respiratory tract is the most common primary site of invasive infection due to inhalation of conidia, but any organ can be affected as part of a primary infection or following dissemination. Aspergillus infection is invasive in immunocompromised subjects, causing disastrous mucosal and bone destruction due to its rapid progression through angioinvasion. The fungal hyphae invade the arteries and form thromboses, reducing the blood supply and causing necrosis of hard and soft tissues. Intracranial and intraorbital extensions are possible in the absence of treatment, putting the vital prognosis at risk. Intracranial involvement following invasion of the frontal sinuses, the cavernous sinus, the carotid artery or the anterior or middle cranial fossa via the cerebral artery is generally fatal and reduces survival, with a mortality rate of 40-80%. (21)

Oral lesions are rarer and may occur through progression of infection from the maxillary sinus, primary infection of the mucosa, direct inoculation following surgery or hematogenous dissemination of the disease from another site, often the lung. (54)

4.2. Exobuccal signs

The patient suffers from headache, pain, fever, facial swelling on the infected side, nasal congestion and purulent rhinorrhea. Sinonasal aspergillosis is usually accompanied by destruction of surrounding structures. It may extend to the orbit and cranial vault, along the base of the skull and large vessels. Symptoms of orbital extension include proptosis, chemosis, ophthalmoplegia and partial or total loss of vision. (48)

4.3. Intra-oral signs

The infection affects the hard palate, the soft palate, the alveolar bone, the bony crevices and the posterior part of the tongue. The palate is often perforated, leading to bucco-sinus or bucco-nasal communication (59).

Intra-oral examination usually reveals **aspergillary osteomyelitis**. (54) Fungal osteomyelitis is most often caused by Candida infection. Aspergillus osteomyelitis is rarer (25).

This is a debilitating and serious form of aspergillosis. It can cause extensive destruction of the soft tissue and bone in the oral cavity. It may be associated with a fistula or diffuse tumour on the infected side, in addition to tooth loss and mobility.

Oral aspergillosis presents two clinicopathological stages. The initial stage reveals isolated, violaceous areas in the gingiva, which may evolve into necrotic, greyish ulcerations. In general, the base of the ulceration shows vascular invasion which may lead in the late stage to the exposure of necrotic bone and mobile bony sequestration which may be attributed to thrombotic vascular infarction and direct tissue destruction (25).

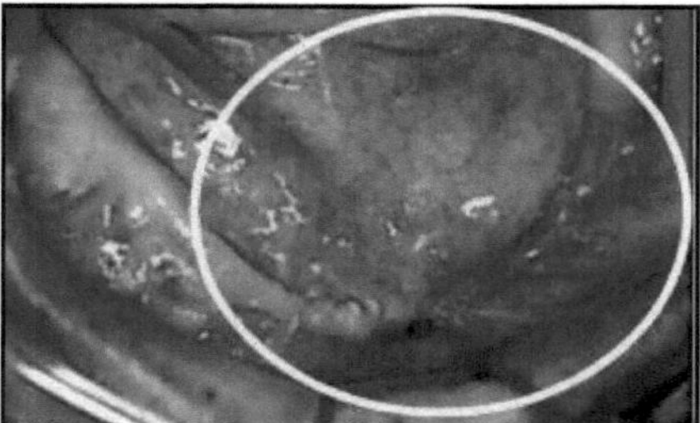

Figure 13. Clinical aspect of oral aspergillosis: fistula and ulceration of the left mucosa (25)

5. Radiological signs of aspergillosis

Panoramic radiography is a screening test for sinus filling and bone destruction.

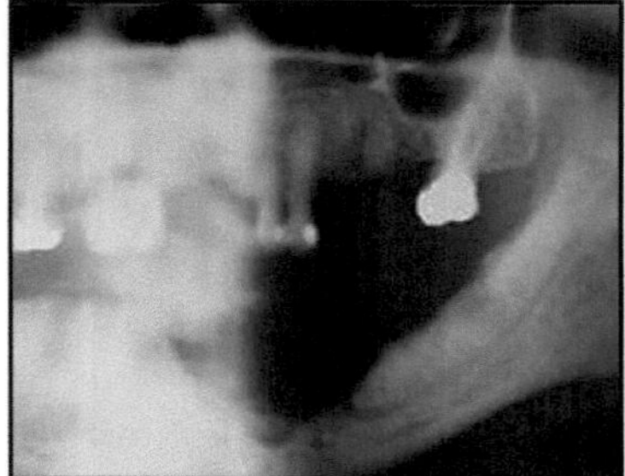

Figure 14. Panoramic radiograph of Aspergillus mandibular osteomyelitis

showing marginal bone resorption with ill-defined margins. (25)

CT and MRI are used to study the extent of the infection in adjacent structures and to assess the severity of the infection. Cross-sectional imaging provides a three-dimensional study of the limits of bone destruction and the filling of air cavities (nasal cavity, maxillary sinus, frontal sinus, etc.). Opacification and hyperdense elements are observed in the infected maxillary sinus. Soft tissue invasion, vascular invasion and involvement are best appreciated on MRI. An increase in T2-weighted MRI signal intensity indicates the presence of an infectious process. Radiological signs are usually discovered late in the clinical course (48).

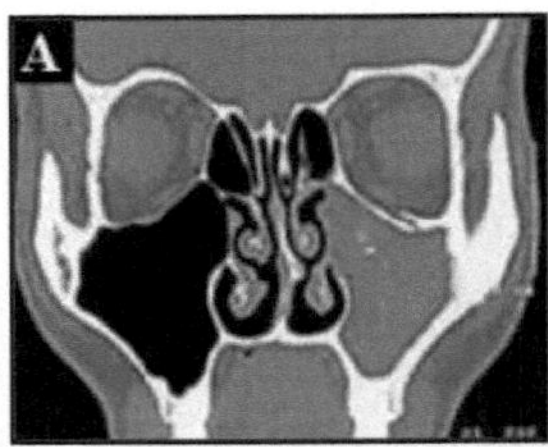

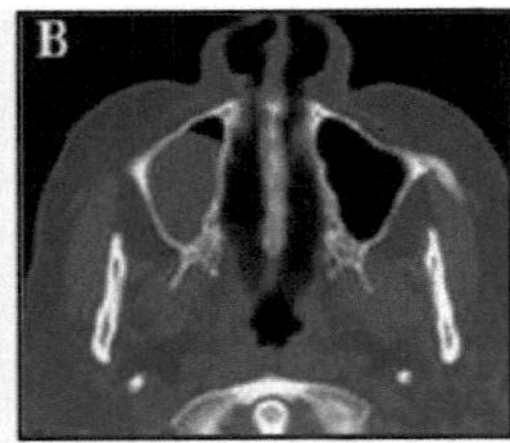

Figure 15. A: frontal section showing the filling of the maxillary sinus, bone lysis and infiltration of the nasal cavity and orbit on the left side (66)
B: axial section showing filling of the right maxillary sinus

The clinico-radiological results can be misleading because the lesions are locally destructive, mimicking a neoplasm and other invasive mycoses, which is why laboratory tests are needed to make a definitive diagnosis.

6. Diagnostic tools

Suspicion may arise in cases of purulent rhinosinusitis that does not respond to antibiotics and on the basis of radiological features. Aspergillosis should be suspected in patients with refractory or recurrent sinusitis.

6.1. Conventional methods

The demonstration of Aspergillus fungal filaments in biopsy tissue samples is an important diagnostic step. Late diagnosis of any invasive infection is associated with a high mortality rate.

6.1.1. Direct microscopic examination

KOH staining of the relevant sinus tissue revealed septate hyphae with dichotomous branching. This diagnosis was confirmed by histopathological examination of the tissues. (66)

6.1.2. Cultivation

Cultures on Sabouraud's dextrose gelose are used to isolate the Aspergillus species and test its sensitivity to antifungal agents, especially in the case of recurrent infection. Cultures are taken at 30 to 37°C for 4 to 5 days, but it is advisable to extend the culture to 7 days, especially if the patient is already on antifungal therapy. However, culture sensitivity is moderate and the turnaround time is long (67).

6.1.3. Histopathological examination

This is the most reliable diagnostic test, but may delay the initiation of treatment. Histopathological examination with specific stains including PAS, GMS and hematoxylin and eosin staining, shows abundant, narrow, septate, typical, aspergillus-specific fungal hyphae with dichotomous branching. While the mucormycosis hyphae are large and nonseptate with open-angle branching, the aspergillus hyphae are septate with 45° branching. Non-caseating granulomatous inflammation, eosinophils and giant cells are also present. The invasive power of the fungi becomes more lethal when the hyphae penetrate the blood vessels and form thrombi (48).

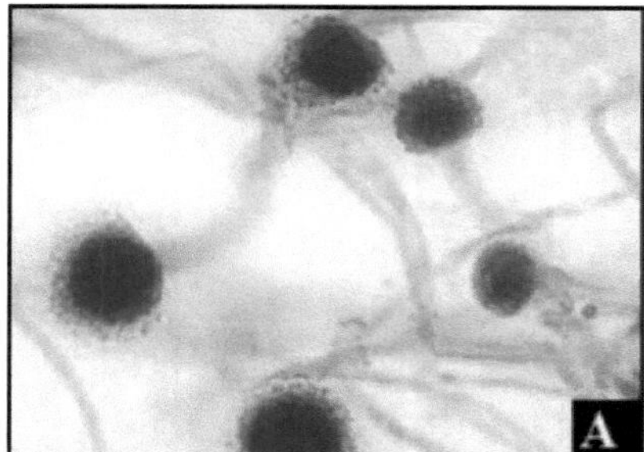

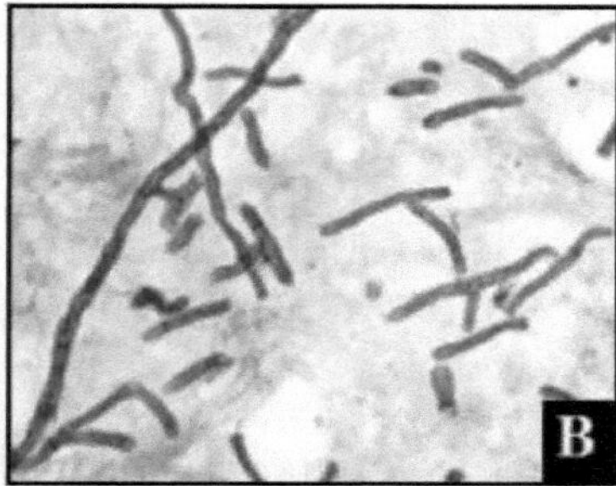

Figure 16. A: Lactophenol blue stain: septate hyphae and coniodophore enlarged at the end forming a tumefied vesicle (48) B: GMS stain showing Aspergillus hyphae narrow and branched at 45° (25)

6.2. Modern methods

Testing for fungal antigens and antibodies appears to be effective.

6.2.1. Detection of galactomannan (GM)

Galactomannan is found in most fungal species except mucorales and Cryptococcus. It is a cell wall polysaccharide released during tissue invasion. A double sandwich enzyme-linked immunosorbent assay uses the monoclonal antibody EB-A2 to detect galactomannan, with a sensitivity of 81%. A new test, Lateral Flow Device (LFD) or aspergillus-specific lateral flow technology, uses the monoclonal antibody JF5 to detect the extracellular mannoproteic antigen secreted exclusively during active aspergillus growth (4).

6.2.2. Detection of (1,3)-Beta-D-glucan

Fungal marker for many fungi, particularly aspergillus (4)

6.2.3. DNA detection by PCR

Molecular tests are alternative options for diagnosing aspergillosis and appear to be promising, although there is a lack of standardisation and wide variation in diagnostic performance (51).

7. Therapeutic methods

A combination of surgical debridement and antifungal therapy.

7.1. Antifungal treatment

Aspergillus is not sensitive to fluconazole, so the latter is ineffective.

Voriconazole (6 mg/kg IV 2 times on 1er day, followed by 4 mg/kg IV 2*/d) is the drug of choice against aspergillosis due to its increased tolerance and efficacy. However, the administration of voriconazole is not free from adverse effects. Prolonged intravenous treatment may cause reversible visual disturbances, increase liver enzymes, alter renal function by accumulation of fluorides or trigger cutaneous epidermoid carcinoma in light-skinned individuals. The concentration of hepatic enzymes should therefore be checked before and during treatment (every 2 to 4 weeks), exposure to the sun should be avoided during treatment and should be avoided in cases of significant renal insufficiency.

Liposomal AMB (5 mg/kg/day IV) is used in 2eme intention or against refractory aspergillosis, although conventional AMB (0.5-1.0 mg/kg) is used as a rescue treatment.

Isavuconazole and posaconazole are effective for aspergillosis, with less hepatic toxicity and fewer drug interactions than voriconazole.

Echinocandins are indicated as part of combined therapy for aspergillosis that is refractory or resistant to azoles.

The optimal duration of antifungal treatment depends on the extent of the disease, the response to treatment and the severity of immunodepression. It varies from 4 weeks to 12 weeks or more (67).

Antifungal prophylaxis: (Itraconazole 400 mg/d or Voriconazole 200 mg*2/d by VO) (9). Antifungal prophylaxis has been shown to be effective against aspergillus and is part of standard care in high-risk patients with prolonged and severe neutropenia, in order to prevent recurrence of the disease (as was the case in our 3eme case report). (77)

7.2. Surgical treatment

This complementary approach to antifungal treatment also improves the response to medical treatment. Early and complete removal of infected necrotic tissue prevents the infection from spreading, thereby reducing morbidity and mortality. Various surgical techniques are used, such as the Caldwell-Luc procedure and endoscopic surgery.

Facial translocation involves temporarily removing the facial bone unit, then re-implanting and fixing it after resection of the lesions -> a beneficial approach in the case of extensive sinus or orbital lesions, improving access to the infected site and avoiding damage to the surrounding vital structures.

Occasionally, surgical resection of the jaw is necessary, resulting in extensive defects that represent a challenge for the surgeon, who must replace not only the avulsed teeth, but also the tissue loss, with a view to restoring function, aesthetics and quality of life, and avoiding psychosocial problems for the patient. (21)

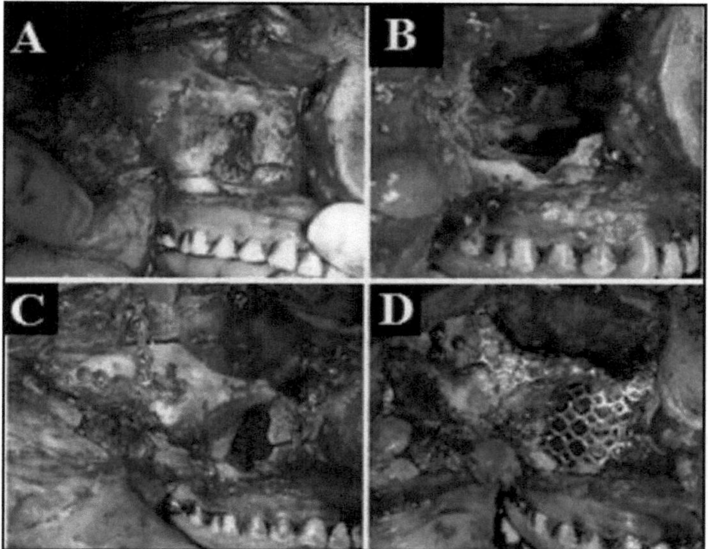

Figure 17. Facial translocation technique: (21) A: Temporary removal of orbito-zygomatico-maxillary bone flap to facilitate access.

B : Debridement of the fungal mass with preservation of the optic nerve
C and D : Bone flap repositioned and reconstruction of the orbital floor and sinus wall

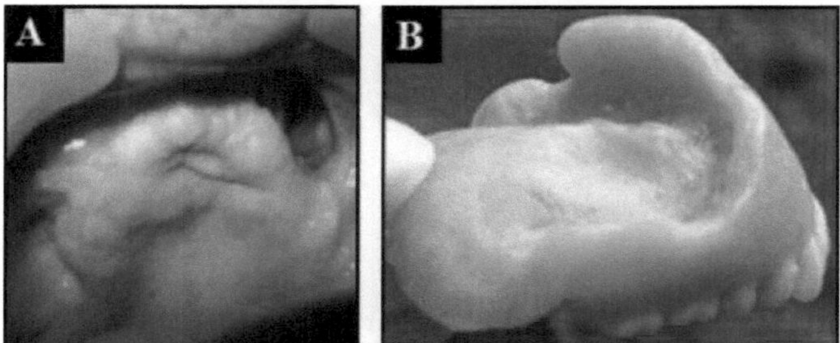

Figure 18. A: formation of a postoperative buccosinusal communication

B : Prosthetic rehabilitation with a complete obturator prosthesis (59)

8. Prognosis

Strongly dependent on the severity of immunodepression and the quality of treatment employed, early diagnosis combined with aggressive treatment initiated as early as possible can improve the prognosis of the disease. Regular clinical, radiological and laboratory follow-up is required for at least 6 months (9).

9. Differential diagnosis

Includes mucormycosis, neoplasms, syphilis, oral tuberculosis, sarcoidosis, Wegener's granulomatosis and allergic fungal sinusitis (54).

10. Coinfection aspergillosis mucormycosis

Concomitant mixed fungal infections exist but are rare. They are invasive and associated with a high mortality rate. In addition to systemic immunodepression, covid-19 is strongly linked to the increased incidence of co-infection, since it is responsible for immune alterations including increased cytokine expression and a decrease in CD4+ and CD8+ T cells.

One mechanism of coinfection is a primary aspergillary infection affecting the sinus or nasal mucosa with invasion of adjacent structures. As the nasal or sinus mucosal tissue was already destroyed by the aspergillary infection, there would have been easy entry of mucorales leading to aspergillosis-mucormycosis co-infection (55). The same diagnostic methods used for isolated infection are indicated for concomitant infection. Histopathology reveals mixed species (aspergillus and mucorales). (14)

Chapter 5

Rare invasive mycoses of the oral cavity

1. Oral cryptococcosis

Caused by Cryptococcus neoformans, which often attacks the immune system. The yeast can remain latent in the phagolysosome for many years. The mucopolysaccharide capsule and other virulence factors (production of melanin, mucin, phospholipase and urease) allow survival in macrophages and tissue propagation of the fungi. Oral cryptococcosis is extremely rare and includes tumefactions, violent nodules, granulomas, draining sinuses, erythematous plaques and oral ulcerations. (10)

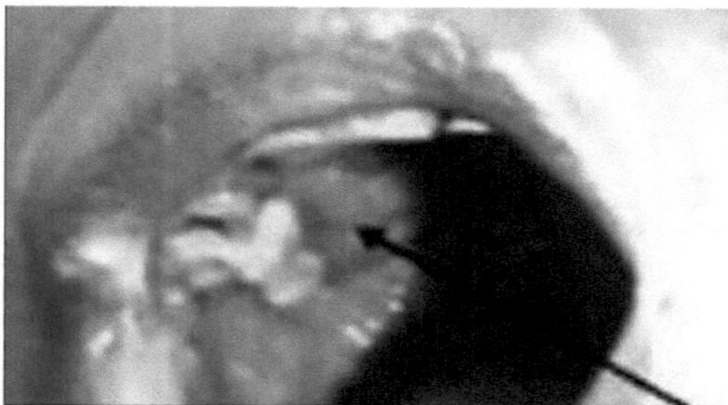

Figure 19. Cryptococcus palatal ulcers with purulent discharge (57)

Histopathology shows multinucleated cells containing micro-organisms of 4 to 6 pm surrounded by a clear halo (the capsule). Fluconazole (400mg) is effective, but AMB is preferred when associated with cryptococcal meningitis or pulmonary involvement. (10)

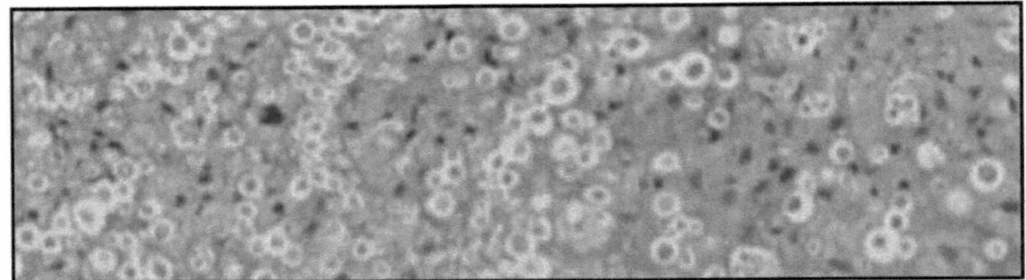

Figure 20. Histological aspect showing the characteristic capsule (0)

2. Oral histoplasmosis

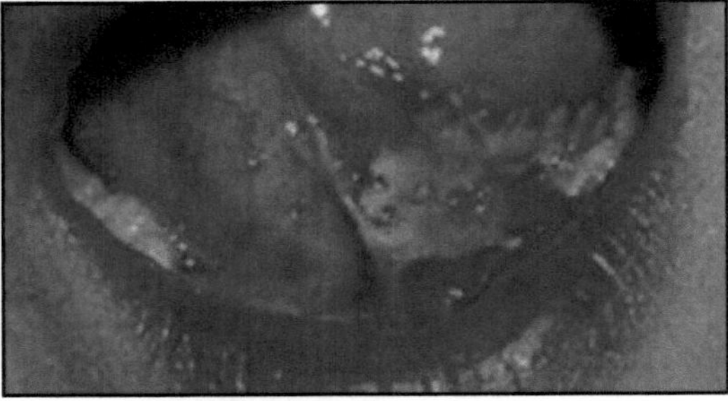

Figure 21. Lingual and floor of mouth ulcerations (3)

This is a deep-seated fungal infection caused by Histoplasma capsulatum. This dimorphic fungal pathogen is found in soils rich in bird and bat droppings. Isolated oral lesions are rare, frequently associated with disseminated or acute pulmonary histoplasmosis^. The endobuccal appearance corresponds to solitary erosions and ulcerations with irregular surfaces and raised, curled margins, covered with a yellow or greyish membrane. Amphotericin B is the initial treatment, followed by itraconazole to prevent recurrence. A poor prognosis is often observed. (53)

3. Oral blastomycosis

Caused by Blastomyces dermatitidis, a dimorphic spore-forming fungus found in acidic, moist, sandy soils. Oral infection is characterised by progressive warty or papular growth or painful ulcerated lesions with hardened, raised margins, which may or may not be associated with osteitis. Histopathology reveals yeast cells 8 to 20 pm in size with double-refractory capsules and attachment of buds to the mother cell. Culture takes two to three weeks. Systemic amphotericin B is the treatment of choice in immunocompromised patients. (10)

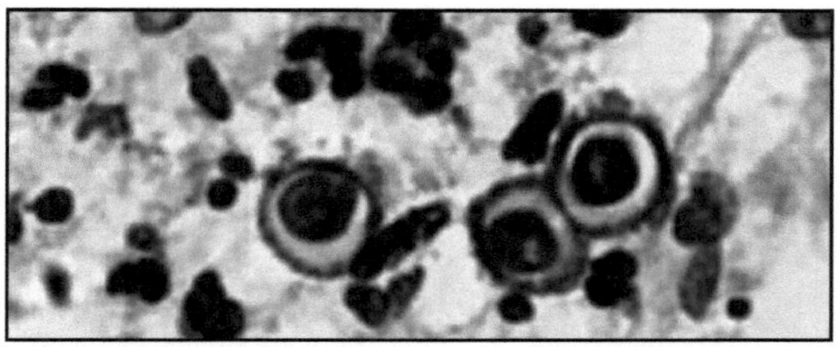

Figure 22. Budding appearance and typical capsule of blastomyces dermatitidis (60)

Chapter 6

Summary table

Infection	Invasive candidiasis	Mucormycosis	Aspergillosis
General	- includes bloodstream infections (candidiasis) and infections deep tissue. - candidemia, the most common. - A deep-rooted disease : osteomyelitis, rhinosinusitis, deep mucocutaneous candidiasis.	- rare but highly aggressive opportunistic infection with a high mortality rate - angioinvasive properties -> thrombus formation -> ischemia and infarction of affected tissue -> tissue necrosis.	- primary sinonasal aspergillosis with or without oral aspergillosis - limited or fulminant (acute) - progresses through the tissue planes with the possibility of vascular invasion
Incidence	+++ most frequent	++	+
etiopathology	Candida albicans ++ and more virulent non-albicans species.	Mucorales: Rhizopus oryzae is the most widely detected.	Aspergillusfumigatus++ Aspergillus flavus +
	- saprophyte in air, water, soil, nutrients and decomposing organic matter. - Transmission by inhalation, ingestion, direct inoculation or dissemination		
Factorsof virulence	Cell adhesion, dimorphism, thermotolerance, capsule presence, enzyme and protein release, iron acquisition.		
Resistance to antifungal agents	- acquired resistance to fluconazole + - C.krusei: intrinsic resistance to fluconazole. - C.glabrata: trend towards resistance to echinocandins.	Resistance to echinocandins.	Trend in azole resistance (fluconazole ++)
Factorsof major risks	-Secondary to any state of	- Diabetemalcontrole ,	- Neutropeniesevereet

	immunodepression -IV drug users, intravenous catheters, malnutrition...	diabetic acidocetosis +++ - Malignant hemopathies ++ - Severe damage caused by covid-19 +.	prolongee (troubles and immunosuppressive therapies)
Exobuccal signs	fever, mouth and/or facial pain, headache, facial swelling on the infected side, nasal congestion, purulent rhinorrhea.		
Extraoral extensions	- to adjacent air cavities (maxillary sinus, frontal sinus, ethmoidal sinus) - extending to the orbit and cranial vault, along the base of the skull and large vessels.		
intraoral signs	- Candidiasis osteomyelitis often of the mandible^ bone exposure necrotic. - Invasive rhinosinusitis: complicated sinusitis with atypical signs. - Deep mucocutaneous candidiasis: varies from papulo-pustular to necrotic plaques.	- Pus discharge, halitosis, tooth mobility, painful necrotic ulcers. - Lesions that are initially red, then purple and finally black^exposed necrotic lesions and sometimes fistulae. - Symptomatology variable rhinosinus.	- often spreads from the maxillary sinus - Diffuse tumefaction of the infected site + tooth mobility and loss, isolated violent areas that progress to greyish necrotic ulcerations, necrotic bone and mobile bone sequences.
Radiological aspects	- CT: to assess the rupture of bony cortices, nasal and/or sinus walls, bone lysis of alveolar processes, filling of air cavities, etc. - MRI better suited to exploring soft tissue extension.		
Conventional diagnostic methods requiring tissue biopsy			
Direct microscopy (KOH)	+	+	+
Histopathology	With specific stains such as Schiff's periodic acid (PAS), hematoxylin-eosin (H&E) or Grocott-Gomori methenamine silver stain (GMS).		
	Hyphae septate or pseudoseptate in	Hyphae wide (5-20 pm), thin-walled,	Narrow, septate hyphae with

	clusters with budding yeast cells in the focal areas. 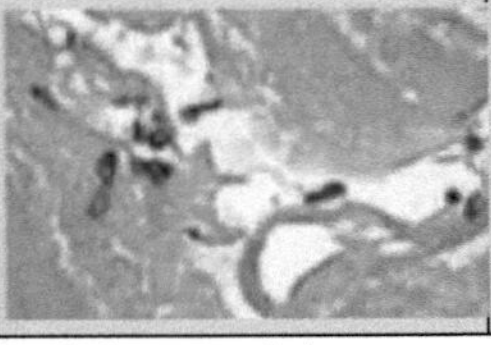	rubanous, not septate, branching at 90°. 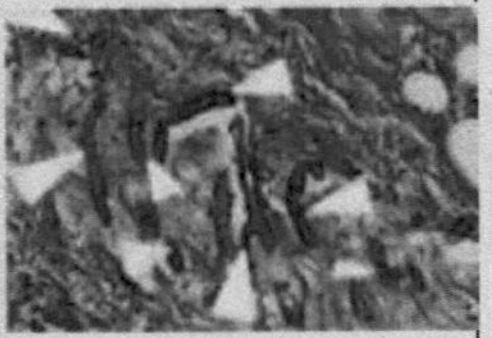	dichotomous branches at 45°. 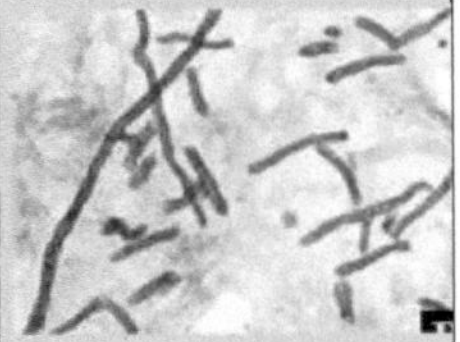
culture	In Sabouraud dextrose gelosis^ isolate the species responsible and test its sensitivity to antifungal agents, especially in the case of recurrent infection.		
	and whitening after 24-48 hours	develops in 3 to 5 days at 2530°C.	between 30 and 37°C for 4 to 5 days
Modern diagnostic methods			
Detection of antigenes or antibodies	mannans, antimannans, в-D- glucan	Mucor fucomannan	galactomannan, в-D-glucan
PCR test	based on nucleic acid amplification^ identify yeasts directly in samples		
Other new products		* Lateral flow test * evaluationofcytokines CD154 POSITIVE	Lateral flow test to detect galactomannan
Treatment			
Surgical treatment	- debridement, curettage, sequestrectomy, sometimes total maxillary resection, complete removal of infected sinuses or aggressive debridement of the retro-orbital space - Rhinosinusitis: medium meatotomy + intrasinus curettage, endoscopy, Caldwell Luc technique... - reconstructive surgery and obturator rehabilitation are often necessary.		
Preferred antifungal treatment	- Fluconazole (Diflucan) 400 mg (6 mg/kg) per day - Liposomal amphotericin B (3 to 5 mg/kg/day): treatment of choice in cases of	- Liposomal AMB (5-10 mg/kg, daily): empirical drug of choice ^ less nephrotoxic but risk of hepatotoxicity	- Voriconazole IV (6 mg/kg*2/d the first day, followed by 4 mg/kg*2 /d) employed with PRECAUTIONS! - Liposomal AMB

	fluconazole resistance or bone involvement.	dose-dependent	(5 mg/kg/d IV)
Other associated therapies	- Hyperbaric oxygen therapy - Elimination of local factors and compliance with treatment of the general disease causing immunodepression. - Oral antifungal prophylaxis in cases of severe and prolonged neutropenia.		
Prognosis	highly dependent on the severity of immunodepression, the virulence of the causative micro-organism, the surgeon's skills, the antifungal molecule chosen and the time at which antifungal treatment is started ^regular follow-up for 2 years or more to prevent recurrence of infection		

Chapter 7

Clinical cases

Here are a few clinical cases that were investigated and treated in our unit of oral medicine and surgery in the dental medicine department at the "farhat hached" university hospital in Sousse, Tunisia.

1. Clinical case N° 1

An 84-year-old patient was admitted to the dermatology department for malnutrition caused by multiple painful ulcerations in the oral cavity that had been developing for 4 days, with no associated skin involvement. The patient was referred to us for an oral examination.

Exobuccal examination revealed a very painful infiltrating black necrotic ulceration covered by crusts 2 cm in width, located in the right labial commissure.

Endobuccal examination revealed deep, necrotizing ulcers in multiple sites: inner surface of the lips, floor of the mouth, posterior surface of the tongue, inner surface of the cheek (retrocommis sural) ...

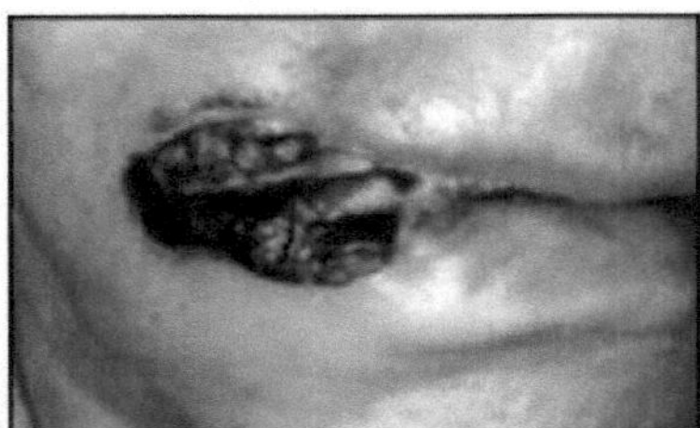

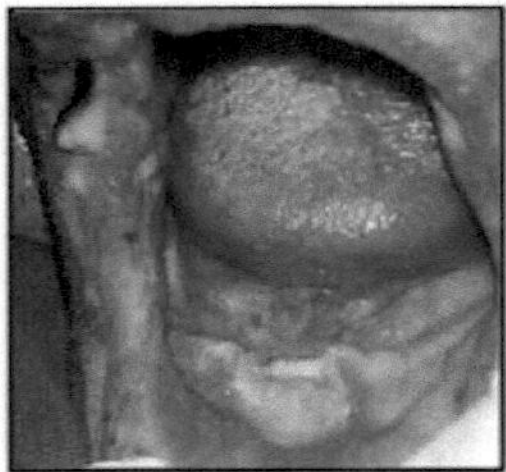

Figure 23. Initial state of the crusty lesion Figure 24. Endobuccal appearance of multiple ulcerations

Biological tests have already been carried out showing :

- Increase in CRP: 145 (normal level < 6mg/L) -^suspicion of inflammatory or infectious syndrome.
- CBC: WBC: 1500 (normal rate between 4,000 and 10,000 WBC/mm3) -^Leukopenia
- PNN: 990 / mcL (normal rate varies from 1,500 to 7,000 / mcL) -^Neutropenia
- HB: 8.8 (12.5 g/ dl for women) -> anemia.
- Platelets: 112,000 with presence of macro-platelets (normal rate between 150,000 and 300,000/mm3) -> thrombocytopenia.

The diagnostic hypotheses put forward were :

a. <u>In relation to the general condition, given the disturbance in the</u> blood <u>count</u>:

1/ Idiopathic pancytopenia (anaemia, thrombocytopenia, neutropenia).

2/ Diffuse malignant haemopathy (lymphoma, leukaemia).

b. In relation to the oral lesions, the diagnostic orientation was towards: Multiple ulcerations caused by saprophytic bacterial flora (streptococci ++) as a result of weakened tissue defence linked to neutropenia.

The initial course of action was as follows

1- Prescription of antibiotics to treat ulcers and prevent bacterial superinfection (amoxicillin/clavulanic acid 2g/d)

2- Local antiseptic treatment (mouthwash with 0.2% Chlorhexidine)

3- Consultation with haematology to investigate the etiology of pancytopenia

4- Removal of crusty lesions on the lips under local anaesthetic to improve healing.

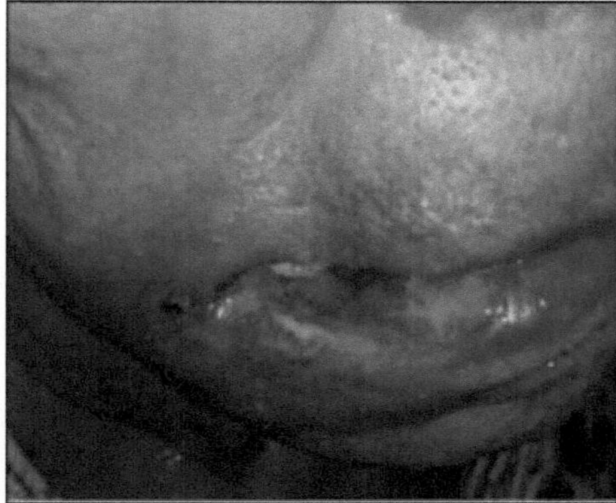

Figure 25. Clinical appearance after stripping of the crust

After 8 days, there was a slight improvement in the endobuccal ulcers.
However, the exobuccal ulceration at the labial commissure had not improved (no healing, intense pain and difficulty eating).

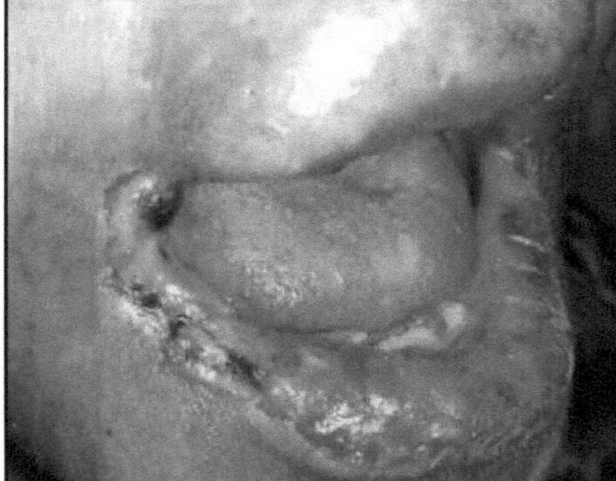

Figure 26. Lack of improvement in the exobuccal lesion after initial therapy

Given the predisposing immunodepression and the presence of neutropenic ulcerations facilitating infiltration of pathogens by rupture of the epithelial barrier, atypical invasive mycotic superinfection was suspected, such as :

- Invasive candidiasis (multi-resistant strain)
- Aspergillosis
- Mucormycosis

The course of action was to carry out :

1. A swab sample for bacteriological and mycological tests.
2. A biopsy with a mycological and anatomopathological examination.
3. A sternal puncture performed in the haematology department for a myelogram.

-> Intermittent pancytopenia was associated with myelodysplastic syndrome.

^ Negative bacteriological examination: massive presence of yeasts with polymorphic flora.

Anatomopathological examination showed deep candidiasis, with typical mycelial filaments revealed by specific PAS and GROCOTT stains.

^ Direct mycological examination: presence of mycelial filaments.

A pathogenic form has been identified in biopsy samples, candida krusei, characterised by its intrinsic resistance to fluconazole and sensitivity to voriconazole -> a common form in neutropenic patients or those on fluconazole prophylaxis.

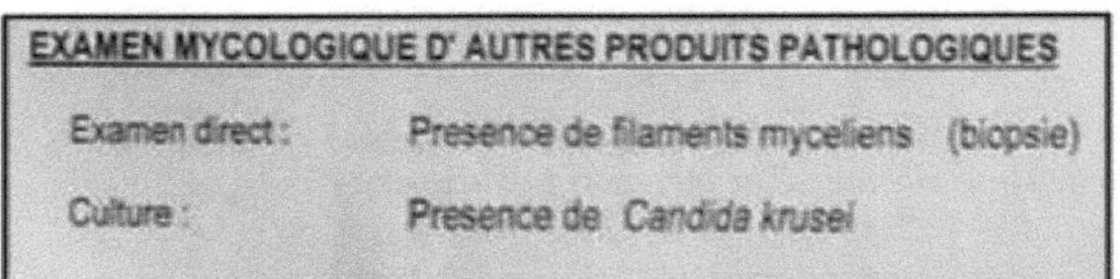
EXAMEN MYCOLOGIQUE D' AUTRES PRODUITS PATHOLOGIQUES

Examen direct :	Presence de filaments myceliens (biopsie)
Culture :	Presence de Candida krusei

Figure 27. Result of mycological examination with detection of Candida krusei

The definitive diagnosis was necrotic ulceration associated with invasive candidiasis caused by candida krusei (favoured by neutropenia).

Suitable treatment: antifungal treatment: voriconazole per os 400mg/d (given immunodepression to prevent the development of other opportunistic mycological infections such as aspergillosis) + hematological management of myelodysplastic syndrome.

2. Clinical case N°2

Patient, 50 years old, diabetic, admitted to the ENT department for possible nasogenous cellulitis evolving for 5 days, was initially treated with a combination of amoxicillin and clavulanic acid 6g/24 h but with no regression.

The patient was referred to the dental medicine department to screen for a possible dental cause. On questioning, the patient emphasised the absence of any initial dental symptoms. The clinical picture was marked by progressive nasolabial swelling, intense left-sided headache and nasal obstruction. The patient also stated that there was no history of chronic maxillary sinusitis.

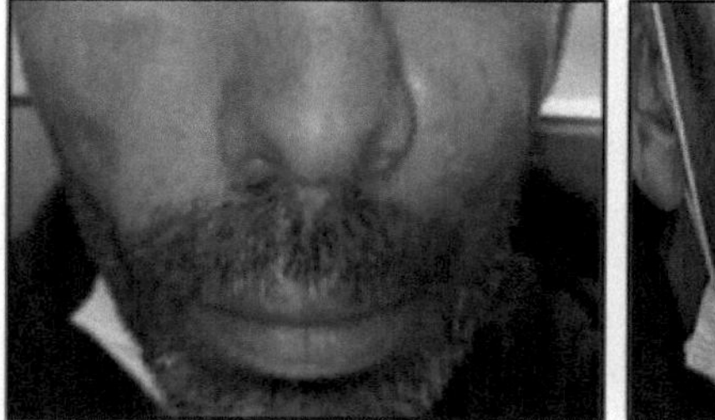
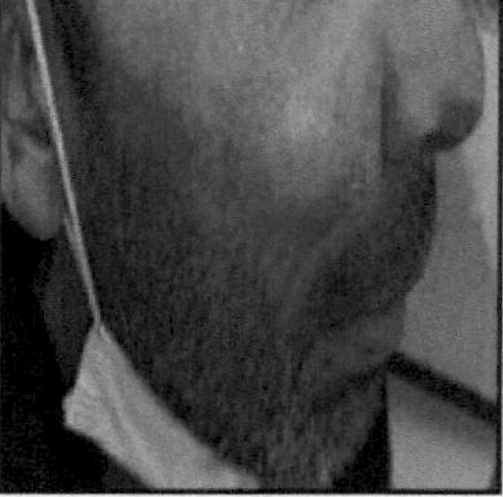

Figure 28. Exobuccal appearance similar to that of left nasolabial cellulitis.

Endobuccal examination revealed :

- Painful palpation of the floor of the vestibule in the premolar edentulous area with no significant filling.
- A negative vitality test on 23 and 24.

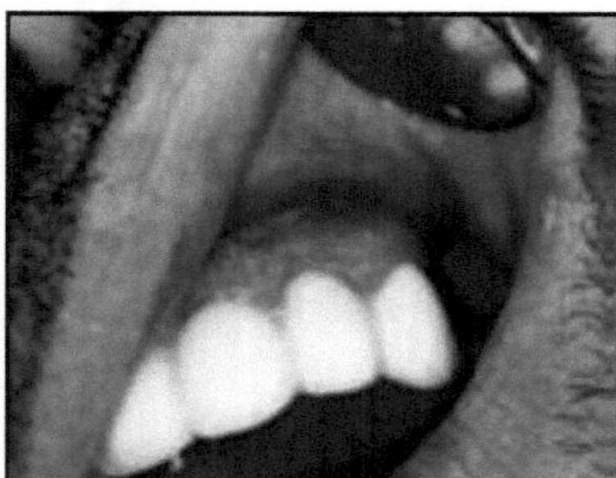

Figure 29. Endobuccal appearance without significant filling

Retroalveolar radiography showed inadequate endodontic treatment of 23 with clinical silence.

Panoramic radiography revealed a left unilateral sinus filling with bone lysis at the sinus floor.

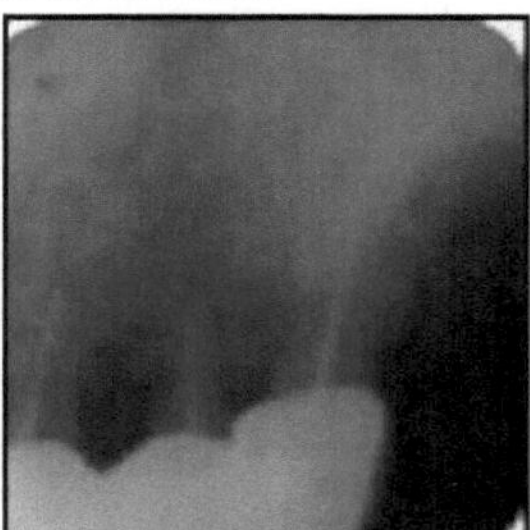
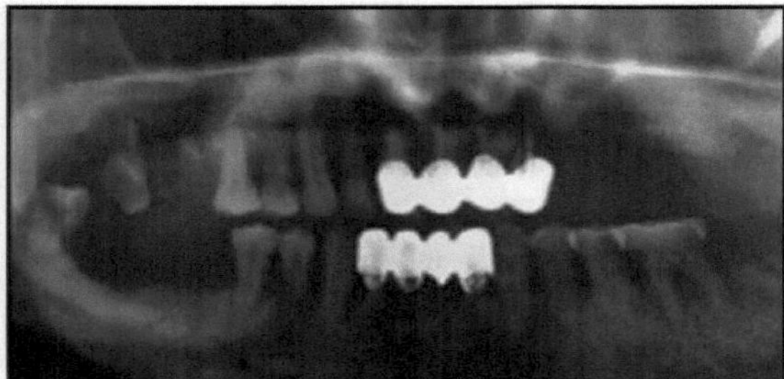

Figure 30. Panoramic radiograph with retroalveolar view shows inadequate endodontic treatment of 23 with radiological silence and left sinus filling.

The hypotheses put forward at this stage:

When the dental examination was negative, the diagnosis of nasolabial cellulitis of dental origin was ruled out (absence of dental symptoms, absence of pain and of filling of the floor of the vestibule opposite the suspect teeth):

1. An invasive fungal infection such as mucormycosis (the patient was diabetic and said he worked in a rural environment as a farmer).

2. Invasive aspergillary maxillary sinusitis.

3. Maxillary osteitis with contiguous reactive sinusitis.

4. Acute bacterial sinusitis of the maxillary rhinus: ruled out if there is genital tumour (a sign of soft tissue invasion), no history of chronic sinusitis and no improvement with antibiotic therapy.

A CT scan of the facial mass was ordered (wide and narrow window) to explore the sinus involvement and associated bone lysis. Two days later, the patient returned with the CT scan. Endobuccal examination revealed the appearance of a left unilateral palatal tumour, with a bluish ischemic appearance of the mucosa and a productive fistula.

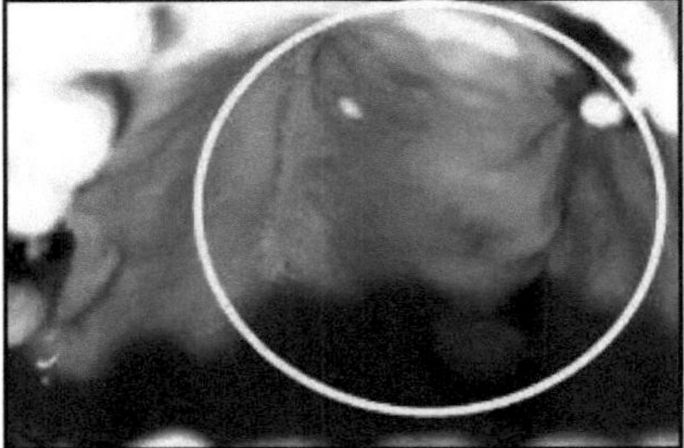

Figure 31. Bluish appearance of the palatal mucosa on the left side and presence of a productive fistula

CT scan: filling of the left maxillary sinus, confinement of the osteomeatal complex, bone lysis in the sinus floor, the medial and anterolateral wall and the lateral aspect of the maxilla.

- > At this stage, on the basis of the clinical and radiological data, the diagnosis of rhinosinus mucormycosis was suggested:
- A diabetic patient from a rural environment with signs of acute invasive maxillary sinusitis (bone lysis of the anterolateral wall and extension into the knee region).
- Recent unilateral palatal tumour with signs of ischaemia and necrosis

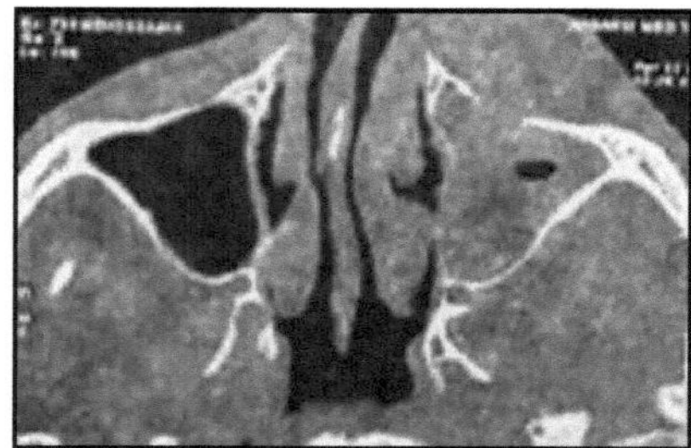

Figure 32. Axial section CT scan in a bone window passing through the middle part of the maxillary sinus. Hyperdense appearance of the left maxillary sinus with bone lysis. of the medial and anterolateral walls.

The treatment was urgent and consisted of :

- A midline meatotomy under endoscopy in the ENT suite, debridement of the left maxillary sinus and biopsy for mycological and anatomopathological examination.
- Infectious disease advice and management to initiate systemic antifungal treatment: liposomal amphotericin B.

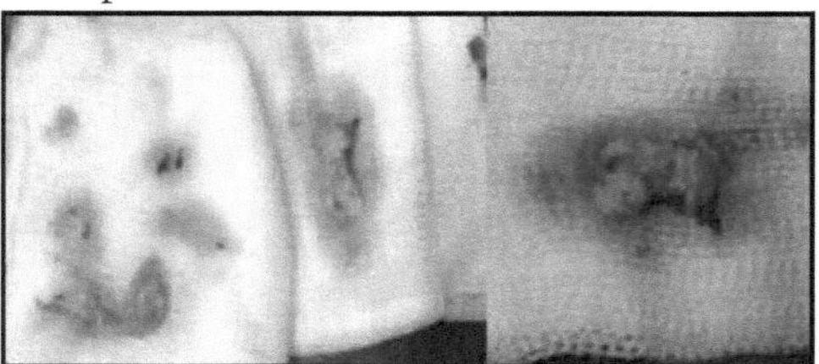

Figure 33. Recovered necrotic debris following medium meatotomy

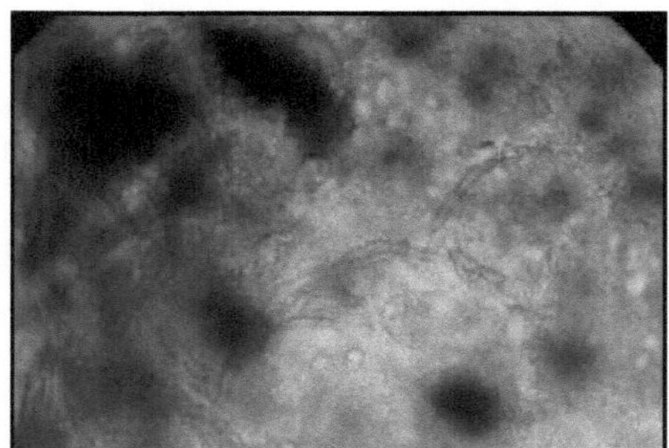

Figure 34. Direct examination under the light microscope: mycelial filaments of Mucorales

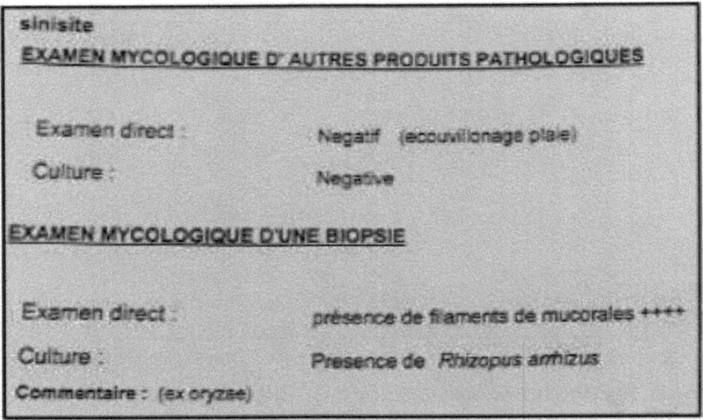
sinisite

EXAMEN MYCOLOGIQUE D' AUTRES PRODUITS PATHOLOGIQUES

Examen direct : Negatif (ecouvillonage plaie)

Culture : Negative

EXAMEN MYCOLOGIQUE D'UNE BIOPSIE

Examen direct : présence de filaments de mucorales ++++

Culture : Presence de *Rhizopus arrhizus*

Commentaire : (ex oryzae)

Figure 35. Result of mycological examination (Rhizopus Arrhizus mucormycosis)

The definitive diagnosis of Rhizopus Arrhizus mucormycosis has been made. Following systemic antifungal treatment (hospitalisation in the infectious diseases department for 3 months), complete resolution of the genital and palatal tumefaction was observed. Early diagnosis of mucormycosis on the basis of oral and dental signs improved the patient's vital prognosis and prevented complications from this invasive mycosis.

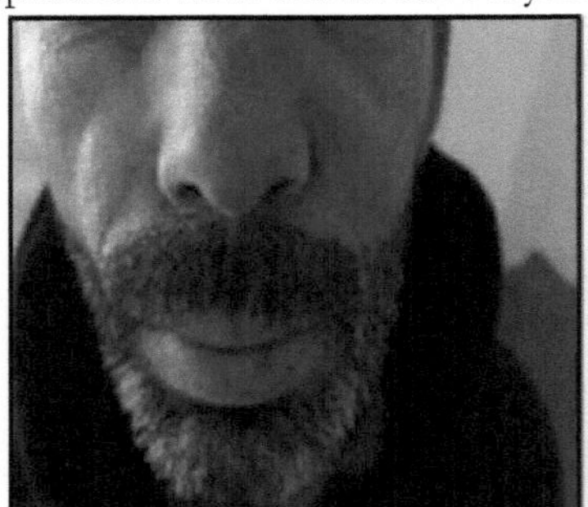
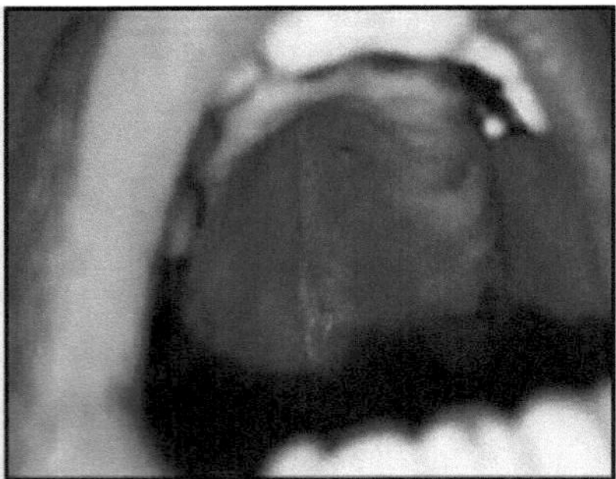

Figure 36. Post-therapeutic exo and endobuccal aspects with disappearance of the exobuccal tumour and normal appearance of the palatal mucosa.

3. Clinical case N°3

Patient H.H, 49 years old, type 2 diabetic, admitted to the ENT department for acute left maxillary sinusitis. She was referred to the dental department in search of a dental etiology.

Exobuccal examination :

Left knee tumour that had been developing for 1 week and was painful to palpation. Endobuccal exaem: slightly violaceous erythematous palatal mucosa on the left side, the second molar is decayed with a negative vitality test.

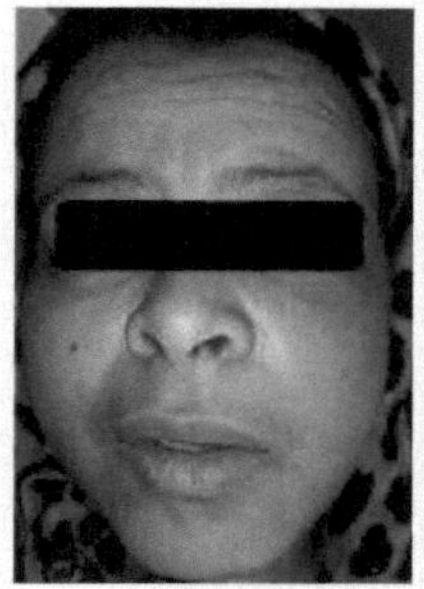

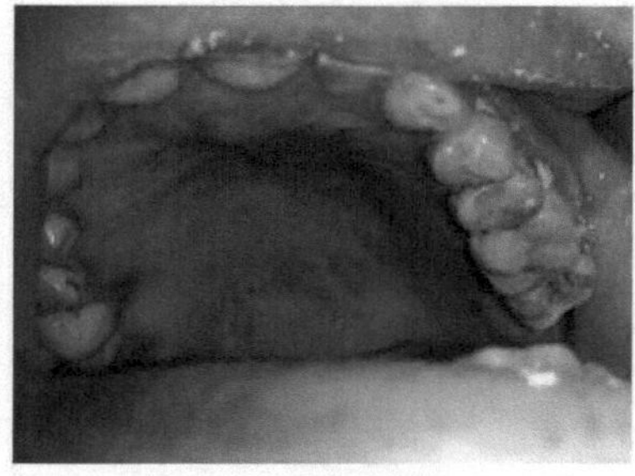

Figure 37. Exobuccal view Figure 38. Endobuccal view

Radiological examination: 27 with adequate endodontic treatment, veil of the Sinus

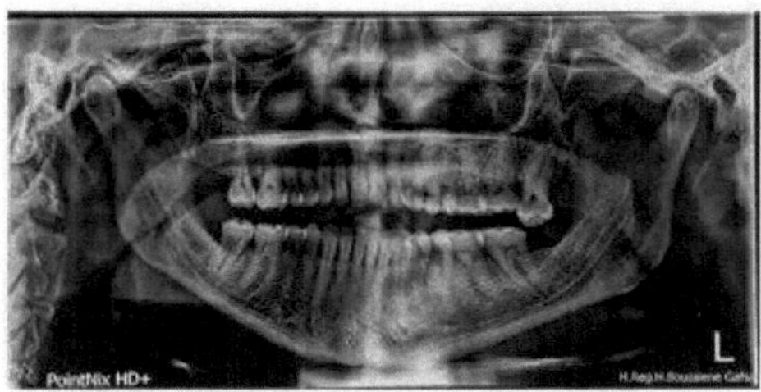

Figure 39. Panoramic radiograph

A CT scan revealed total filling of the left maxillary sinus, with confinement of the osteo meatal complex and filling of the ethmoidal cells. The diagnosis was in favour of chronic reheated maxillary sinusitis associated with chronic apical periodontitis of the 27

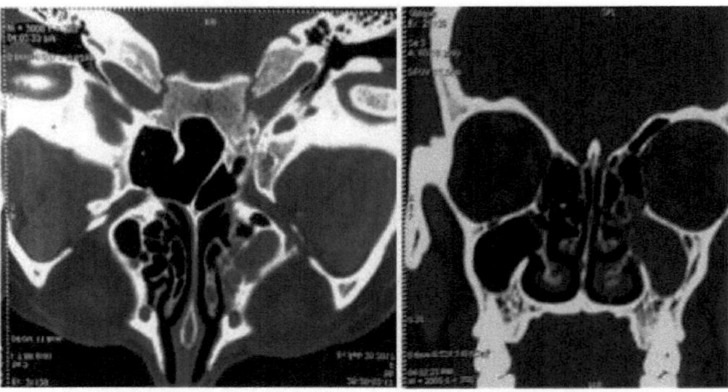

Figure 40. CT axial and frontal section: filling of the maxillary sinus guache

CAT: Overture of the tooth: root canal trimming and provisional obturation, sinus aspiration lavage

Probist antibiotic treatment: amoxicillin/clavulamic acid 3g/d 13d

Evolution: check-up after 5 days: no improvement in rhinological symptoms
The patient returned with a purulent discharge from the sulcus of the posterior teeth, with significant mobility and gingival ulceration.
Suggested diagnosis: invasive fungal infection such as aspergillosis or mucormucosis, given the patient's immunocompromised condition.

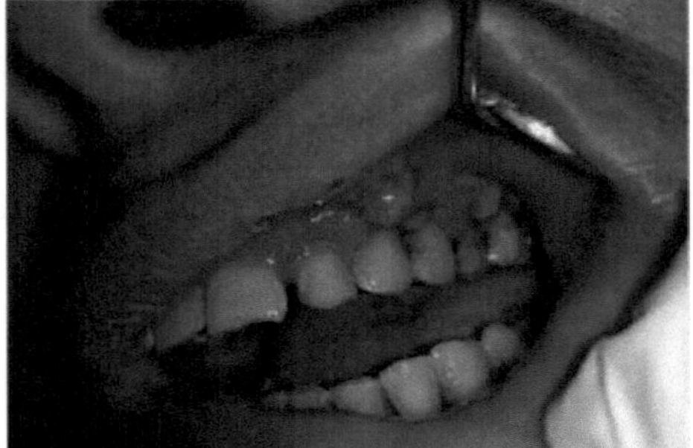

Figure 41. Endobuccal view of the side of the infection

Procedure: midline meatotomy by endoscopy in the operating theatre under general anaesthetic, washing of the sinus and sampling of the sinus mucosa for direct examination and anatomopathological examination.

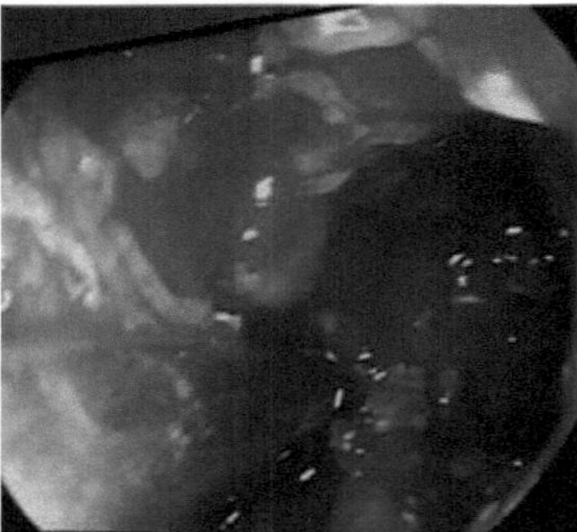

Figure 42. Endoscopic view of the inflamed middle meat

Mycological examination revealed mycelial filaments typical of mucorale.
Anatomopathological examination was positive with PAS staining ++++ confirming the diagnosis of an atypical presentation of rhinosinus mucormycosis. The patient was admitted to the infectious medicine department for administration of liposomal amphotericin B with progressive improvement after one month.

4. Clinical case N°4

A 13-year-old boy, admitted to the haematology department for acute lymphoblastic leukaemia, was a candidate for a bone marrow allograft. He presented with febrile neutropenia, PNN 0. During hospitalisation, the patient developed a painful inflammatory left mandibular tumefaction with no signs of suppuration, diagnosed as genital cellulitis of dental origin.

Given the patient's condition, dental consultation was impossible (patient in severe aplasia) and probabilistic treatment was instituted: broad-spectrum antibiotic therapy, voriconazole 200 mg/d, with no improvement.

Regression of the lower genital tumour was spontaneous and progressive with hematological recovery. The child was referred to the dental medicine department in search of a possible dental etiology.

Endobuccal examination revealed :

- The greyish ischemic appearance of the vestibular mucosa opposite 37, with bone exposure at the neck and septum 37-36.
- No progressive caries on 36 and 37 with positive pulp vitality tests, the retroalveolar click showed desmodontal enlargement of 37.
- Palpation of the floor of the vestibule with pain and no filling opposite the 37.
- Periodontal probing of 37 revealed a vestibular bone sequestrum that was mobile but not detachable.

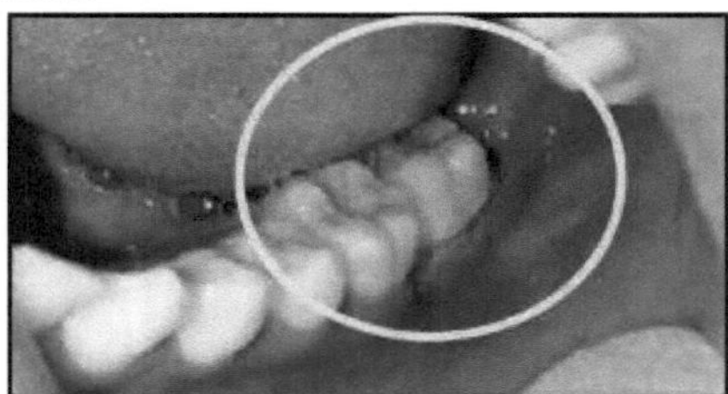

Figure 43. Clinical appearance on endobuccal examination with the presence of a sequestrum vestibular bone.

A mandibular Cone beam **radiological examination** was requested to explore the underlying bone damage: to look for radiological signs of chronic osteitis. Axial and sagittal sections showed a vestibular bone sequestration opposite the 37 with desmodontal widening.

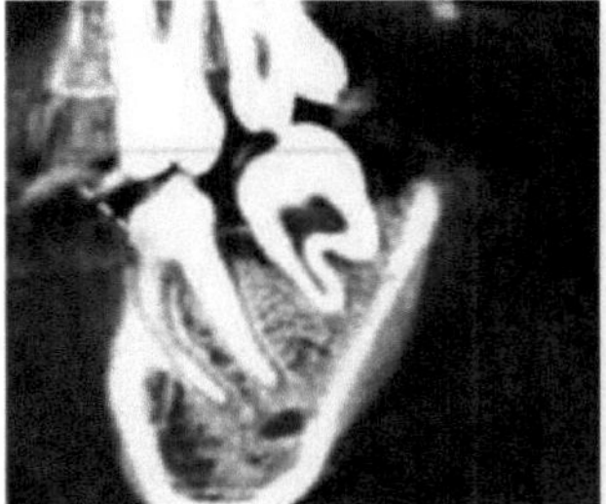

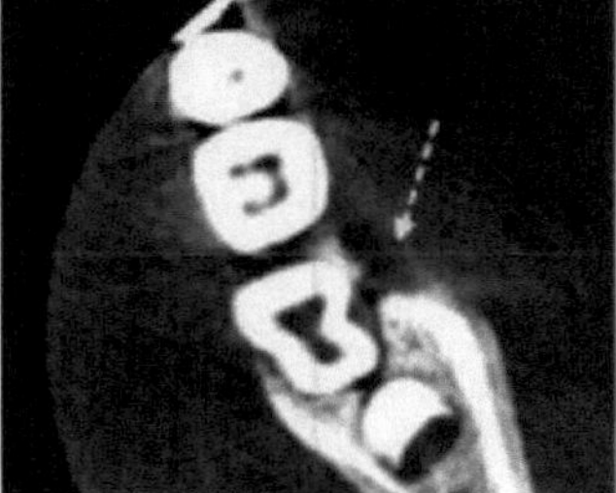

Figure 44. Axial and sagittal sections of the cone beam examination: destruction of the bone cortices opposite 37 and 36

Possible diagnostic hypotheses at this stage: neutropenic ulcerations (during the previous episode of severe neutropenia) complicated by :

1. Non-specific bacterial osteitis

2. Specific osteitis: mycotic, aspergillary or mucosal superinfection (immunocompromised patients).

Treatment was initially surgical, with debridement of the bone, removal of the sequestrum and inflammatory tissue, and biopsy for pathological examination.

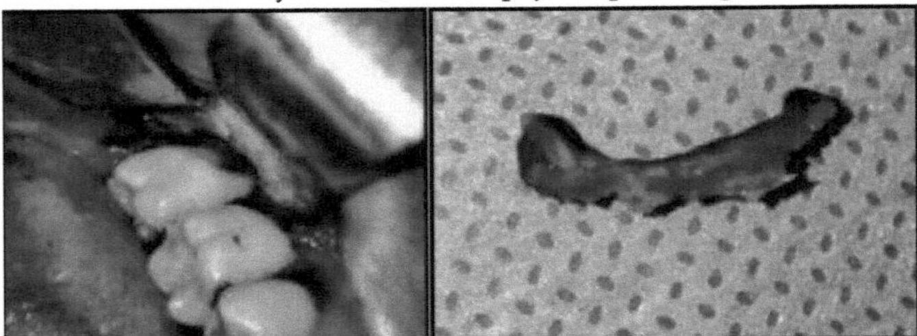

Figure 45. Intraoperative appearance after bone curettage and removal of vestibular bone sequestration

Pathological examination showed a chronic inflammatory remodelling: a polymorphous inflammatory infiltrate, vascular neoformation with aspergillus mycelial filaments present only in the bone sequestrum. **A definitive diagnosis** of chronic aspergillosis was made.

Antifungal treatment was instituted: prescription of voriconazole 100mg/d for 3 months, combined with antibiotic therapy and antiviral treatment (tritherapy) **^ A** patient undergoing allogeneic stem cell transplantation with a risk of recurrence during the deep and prolonged phases of aplasia.

Mucosal healing 15 days after surgical debridement was satisfactory, with complete resolution of pain.

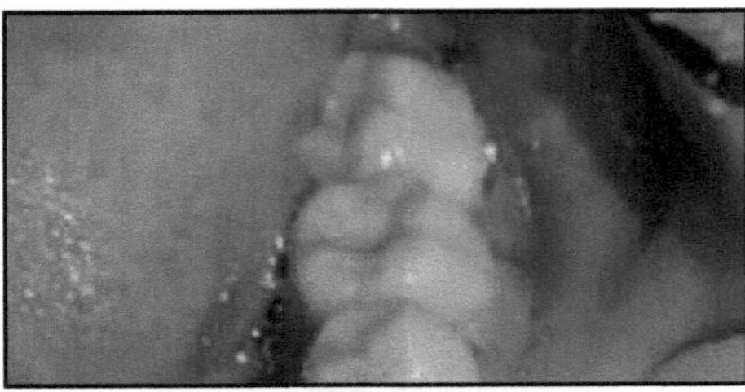

Figure 46. Satisfactory mucosal healing at 15 days post-op.

Aspergillosis is usually invasive and locally destructive. The benign course in this patient was explained by initial antifungal prophylaxis (voriconazole 200 mg/d), confirming the efficacy of this preventive protocol for invasive aspergillosis in immunocompromised patients with medullary aplasia.

Conclusion

A variety of fungal species occupy our environment silently (in a saprophytic state) and wait for a signal (immunodepression) to attack, grow, cause and develop as invasive infections. They are capable of altering any organ, causing deep and locally devastating destruction of mucous and bone structures, disseminating and putting the patient's vital prognosis at risk. Today, an increase in the incidence of invasive fungal infections is strongly associated with an increase in immunodepressive states, resistance to antifungal agents and fungal virulence factors favoured by immunodepression.

Candidiasis is the most common. In immunocompromised patients, Candida tends to cause invasive disease in the form of osteomyelitis, invasive rhinosinusitis, deep mucocutaneous candidiasis or candidemia. Mucorales and aspergillus are quite virulent due to their angioinvasive properties, leading to thrombosis, infarction and tissue necrosis, with rapid progression to neighbouring structures and hematogenic dissemination. Mucormycosis is strongly associated with poorly controlled diabetes. The dominant risk factor associated with aspergillosis is severe and prolonged neutropenia.

Generally, the clinical signs are highly suggestive (ulceration, exposure of necrotic bone, purulent discharge, etc.) and do not respond to antibiotics, suggesting a fungal infection as a differential diagnosis. In some cases, in the early stages of the disease, the practitioner may note discrete orofacial signs, which may nonetheless point towards a diagnosis of invasive mycosis. However, the rhinosinus and/or buccal manifestations can lead to confusion with other conditions such as chronic maxillary osteitis, sinusitis of dental origin and low-grade intraosseous tumours.

Histopathology is a vital diagnostic test, as is culture, to identify the species involved and help choose the right antifungal agent, in addition to new, simpler and faster complementary diagnostic methods. Treatment is based on surgical intervention, sometimes requiring extensive tissue sacrifices, and antifungal therapy. Because of the tendency of fungi to develop resistance to azoles, liposomal amphotericin B, a broad-spectrum drug, is now defined as the treatment of choice for invasive mycoses. The earlier the diagnosis and treatment, the more limited the tissue invasion, the fewer the post-surgical sequelae and the lower the morbidity and mortality rates, which is why knowledge of the clinical and radiological signs of these invasive fungal infections is vital.

References

1. **Afkhamnejad ER, Turner C, Reynoso D.**
A case of orbital cryptococcosis.
Am J Ophthalmol Case Rep 2023;30:1-4.
2. **Angiolella L.**
Virulence regulation and drug-resistance mechanism of fungal infection.
Microorganisms 2022;10(2):1-5.
3. **Anitha KP.**
Fungal infections of the oral mucosa.
Indian J Dent Res 2012;23(5):650-9.
4. **Arastehfar A, Carvalho A, Houbraken J et al.**
Aspergillus fumigatus and aspergillosis: From basics to clinics.
Stud Mycol 2021;100:1-51.
5. **Arias F, Mata-Essayag S, Landaeta ME et al.**
Candida albicans osteomyelitis: Case report and literature review.
Int J Infect Dis 2004;8(5):307-14.
6. **Bali R, Sharma P, Gupta P, Gaba S.**
Chronic candidal osteomyelitis of mid face: A therapeutic dilemma.
J Oral Biol Craniofac Res 2013;3(3):151-3.
7. **Berbudi A, Rahmadika N, Tjahjadi AI, Ruslami R.**
Type 2 diabetes and its impact on the immune system.
Curr Diabetes Rev 2020;16(5):442-9.
8. **Bhandari S, Agarwal S, Bhargava S et al.**
Post Covid-19 Sinonasal candidiasis: A crisis within the pandemic.
Indian J Otolaryngol Head Neck Surg 2023;75(2):523-8.
9. **Bhandari S, Gupta S, Bhargava S et al.**
COVID Associated Invasive Aspergillosis.
Indian J Otolaryngol Head Neck Surg 2023;75(2):557-62.
10. **Bose D, Brizuela M.**
Fungal Infections of the Oral Mucosa.
Treasure Island: StatPearls Publishing, 2023.
11. **Chandra A, Firth J, Sheikh A, Patel P.**
Emergencies related to HIV infection and treatment (part 2): Emergencies related to HIV infection and treatment (part 2).
Afr J Emerg Med 2013;3(4):197-202.
12. **Chavda VP, Mishra T, Kamaraj S et al.**
Post-COVID-19 Fungal Infection in the Aged Population.
Vaccines 2023;11(3):1-26.
13. **Cheng T, Li Y, Zhang H et al.**
Incidence of oral candidiasis is associated with inhaled corticosteroids in

Chinese patients: A systematic review and meta-analysis.
Int J Clin Exp Med 2017;10(3):5546-60.

14. Chugh A, Pandey AK, Goyal A et al.
Atypical presentations of fungal osteomyelitis during post COVID-19 outbreak - case series.
J Oral Maxillofac Surg Med Pathol 2022;34(5):622-7.

15. Coronado-Castellote L, Jimenez-Soriano Y.
Clinical and microbiological diagnosis of oral candidiasis.
J Clin Exp Dent 2013;5(5):279-86.

16. Cortez JL, Tan SY, Abelman R et al.
Deep cutaneous candidiasis of the lip in a patient with acute myelogenous leukemia.
JAAD Case Rep 2022;27:32-4.

17. Dachlan I, Wicaksana A, Fauzi AR et al.
Invasive maxillary aspergillosis in a patient with systemic lupus erythematosus: Case report.
Ann Med Surg 2020;58:44-7.

18. Darwish RM, AlMasri M, Al-Masri MM.
Mucormycosis: The hidden and forgotten disease.
J Appl Microbiol 2022;132(6):4042-57.

19. Deepa A, Nair BJ, Sivakumar T, Joseph AP.
Uncommon opportunistic fungal infections of oral cavity: A review.
J Oral Maxillofac Pathol 2014;18(2):235-43.

20. Dewan H, Patel H, Pandya H, Bhavsar B, Shah U, Singh S.
Mucormycosis of jaws - literature review and current treatment protocols.
Natl J Maxillofac Surg 2022;13(2):180-9.

21. Dhirawani R, Asrani S, Pathak S, Sharma A.
Facial translocation approach for management of invasive sinonasal aspergillosis.
J Maxillofac Oral Surg 2015;14(1):482-7.

22. D^az-Tejedor A, Lorenzo-Mohamed M, Puig N et al.
Immune system alterations in multiple myeloma: Molecular mechanisms and therapeutic strategies to reverse immunosuppression.
Cancers 2021;13(6):1-26.

23. Dimopoulos G, Karabinis A, Samonis G, Falagas ME.
Candidemia in immunocompromised and immunocompetent critically ill patients: A prospective comparative study.
Eur J Clin Microbiol Infect Dis 2007;26(6):377-84.

24. Ekmekciu I, Von Klitzing E, Fiebiger U et al.
Immune responses to broad-spectrum antibiotic treatment and fecal microbiota transplantation in Mice.

Front Immunol 2017;8:1-19.
25. Faustino ISP, Ramos JC, Mariz BALA et al.
A rare case of mandibular aspergillus osteomyelitis in an immunocompetent patient.
Dent J 2022;10(11):1-8.
26. Gamaletsou MN, Kontoyiannis DP, Sipsas NV et al.
Candida osteomyelitis: analysis of 207 pediatric and adult cases (1970-2011).
Clin Infect Dis 2012;55(10):1338-51.
27. Garcia-Hermoso D.
Microbiological diagnosis of mucormycosis.
Med Sci 2013;29:13-8.
28. Gomes MZ, Lewis RE, Kontoyiannis DP.
Mucormycosis caused by unusual mucormycetes, non-Rhizopus, -Mucor, and -Lichtheimia species.
Clin Microbiol Rev 2011;24(2):411-45.
29. Hedayati MT, Pasqualotto AC, Warn PA, Bowyer P, Denning DW.
Aspergillus flavus: Human pathogen, allergen and mycotoxin producer.
Microbiology 2007;153(6):1677-92.
30. Kaushal D, Sharma A, Kesarwani A, Kalita JM.
Chronic Candida osteomyelitis of hard palate and nose: A diagnostic quandary.
Med Mycol Case Rep 2019;24:1-4.
31. Kohler JR, Hube B, Puccia R, Casadevall A, Perfect JR.
Fungi that infect humans.
Microbiol Spectr 2017;5(3):1-29.
32. Kullberg BJ, Arendrup MC.
Invasive candidiasis.
N Engl J Med 2015;373(15):1445-56.
33. Lalla RV, Latortue MC, Hong CH et al.
A systematic review of oral fungal infections in patients receiving cancer therapy.
Support Care Cancer 2010;18(8):985-92.
34. Leventakos K, Lewis RE, Kontoyiannis DP.
Fungal infections in leukemia patients: How do we prevent and treat them?
Clin Infect Dis 2010;50(3):405-15.
35. Li CX, Gong ZC, Pataer P, Shao B, Fang C.
A retrospective analysis for the management of oromaxillofacial invasive mucormycosis and systematic literature review.
BMC Oral Health 2023;23(1):1-28.
36. Li Z, Denning DW.
The impact of corticosteroids on the outcome of fungal disease: A systematic review and meta-analysis.

Curr Fungal Infect Rep 2023;17(1):54-70.
37. Lin SJ, Schranz J, Teutsch SM.
Aspergillosis case-fatality rate: systematic review of the literature.
Clin Infect Dis 2001;32(3):358-66.
38. Little JS, Weiss ZF, Hammond SP.
Invasive fungal infections and targeted therapies in hematological malignancies.
J Fungi 2021;7(12):1-21.
39. Logan A, Wolfe A, Williamson JC.
Antifungal resistance and the role of new therapeutic agents.
Curr Infect Dis Rep 2022;24(9):105-16.
40. Mushi MF, Mtemisika CI, Bader O et al.
High Oral Carriage of Non-albicans Candida spp. among HIV-infected individuals.
Int J Infect Dis 2016;49:185-8.
41. Nouraei H, Jahromi MG, Jahromi LR, Zomorodian K, Pakshir K.
Potential pathogenicity of candida species isolated from oral cavity of patients with diabetes mellitus.
Biomed Res Int 2021;2021:1-6.
42. Okoye CA, Nweze E, Ibe C.
Invasive candidiasis in Africa, what is the current picture?
Pathog Dis 2022;80(1):1-17.
43. Pai V, Sansi R, Kharche R, Bandili SC, Pai B.
Rhino-orbito-cerebral mucormycosis: Pictorial review.
Insights Imaging 2021;12(1):1-17.
44. Pappas PG, Lionakis MS, Arendrup MC, Ostrosky-Zeichner L, Kullberg BJ.
Invasive candidiasis.
Nat Rev Dis Primers 2018;4(1):1-20.
45. Paramythiotou E, Frantzeskaki F, Flevari A, Armaganidis A, Dimopoulos G.
Invasive fungal infections in the ICU: How to approach, how to treat.
Molecules 2014;19(1):1085-119.
46. Patil S, Majumdar B, Sarode SC, Sarode GS, Awan KH.
Oropharyngeal candidosis in HIV-infected patients-an update.
Front Microbiol 2018;9:1-9.
47. Patil S, Rao RS, Majumdar B, Anil S.
Clinical appearance of oral candida infection and therapeutic strategies.
Front Microbiol 2015;6:1-10.
48. Peral-Cagigal B, Redondo-Gonzalez LM, Verrier-Hernandez A.
Invasive maxillary sinus aspergillosis: A case report successfully treated with voriconazole and surgical debridement.

J Clin Exp Dent 2014;6(4):448-51.
49. Prasannasrinivas D, Guledgud MV, Karthikeya P, D'Souza RS.
A non-healing ulcer with unilateral facial palsy.
Br J Med Res 2015 9(5):1-7.
50. Quindos G, Gil-Alonso S, Marcos-Arias C et al.
Therapeutic tools for oral candidiasis: Current and new antifungal drugs.
Med Oral Patol Oral Cir Bucal 2019;24(2):172-80.
51. Quindos G.
New microbiological techniques for the diagnosis of invasive mycoses caused by filamentous fungi.
Clin Microbiol Infect 2006;12:40-52.
52. Rafat Z, Sasani E, Salimi Y, Hajimohammadi S, Shenagari M, Roostaei D.
The prevalence, etiological agents, clinical features, treatment, and diagnosis of HIV-associated oral candidiasis in pediatrics across the world: A systematic review and meta-analysis.
Front Pediatr 2021;9:1-12.
53. Rajendra Santosh AB, Muddana K, Bakki SR.
Fungal infections of oral cavity: Diagnosis, management, and association with COVID-19.
SN Compr Clin Med 2021;3(6):1373-84.
54. Rallis G, Gkinis G, Dais P, Stathopoulos P.
Visual loss due to paranasal sinus invasive aspergillosis in a diabetic patient.
Ann Maxillofac Surg 2014;4(2):247-50.
55. Ramani P, Krishnan RP, Pandiar D, Benitha JG, Ramalingam K, Gheena S.
Chronic invasive aspergillosis with fulminant mucormycosis sparing palate in a Post-COVID-19 patient - a case report.
Ann Maxillofac Surg 2022;12(1):102-5.
56. Rapidis AD.
Orbitomaxillary mucormycosis (zygomycosis) and the surgical approach to treatment: perspectives from a maxillofacial surgeon.
Clin Microbiol Infect 2009;15:98-102.
57. Reyes AJ, Ramcharan K, Aboh S, Giddings SL.
Primary oral cryptococcosis in an HIV-positive woman with suppressed viral load and normal CD4 count: A rare case.
BMJ Case Rep 2021;14(6):1.
58. Robitaille C, Fleury M.
Candida infections: Treatment with oral antifungals.
Med Quebec 2011;46(2):73-5.

59. Rudagi BM, Halli R, Kalburge J, Joshi M, Munde A, Saluja H.
Management of maxillary aspergillosis in a patient with diabetic mellitus followed by prosthetic rehabilitation.
J Maxillofac Oral Surg 2010;9(3):297-301.
60. Saccente M, Woods GL.
Clinical and laboratory update on blastomycosis.
Clin Microbiol Rev 2010;23(2):367-81.
61. Scheinberg P.
Aplastic anemia: therapeutic updates in immunosuppression and transplantation.
Hematology Am Soc Hematol Educ Program 2012;2012:292-300.
62. Segal BH, Walsh TJ.
Current approaches to diagnosis and treatment of invasive aspergillosis.
Am J Respir Crit Care Med 2006;173(7):707-17.
63. SeyedAlinaghi S, Karimi A, Barzegary A et al.
Mucormycosis infection in patients with COVID-19: A systematic review.
Health Sci Rep 2022;5(2):529.
64. Shariati A, Moradabadi A, Chegini Z, Khoshbayan A, Didehdar M.
An overview of the management of the most important invasive fungal infections in patients with blood malignancies.
Infect Drug Resist 2020;13:2329-54.
65. Shetty L, Kulkarni D, Gupta AA, Gawande B.
Maxillary osteomyelitis with candidiasis due to extraction in uncontrolled diabetes state-a case report.
Dentistry 2015;5(2);1-4.
66. Shetty S, Shilpa C, Kavya S, Sundararaman A, Hegde K, Madhan S.
Invasive aspergillosis of nose and paranasal sinus in COVID-19 convalescents: Mold goes viral?
Indian J Otolaryngol Head Neck Surg 2022;74(2):3239-44.
67. Sigera LSM, Denning DW.
Invasive aspergillosis after renal transplantation.
J Fungi 2023;9(2):1-12.
68. Sitheeque MA, Samaranayake LP.
Chronic hyperplastic candidosis/candidiasis (candidal leukoplakia).
Crit Rev Oral Biol Med 2003;14(4):253-67.
69. Struck MF, Gille J.
Fungal infections in burns: a comprehensive review.
Ann Burns Fire Disasters 2013;26(3):147-53.
70. Suresh A, Joshi A, Desai AK et al.
Covid-19-associated fungal osteomyelitis of jaws and sinuses: An experience-driven management protocol.

Med Mycol 2022;60(2):1-9.

71. Swain SK, Sahu MC, Baisakh MR.
Mucormycosis of the head and neck.
Apollo Med 2018;15(1):6-10.

72. Taylor M, Brizuela M, Raja A.
Oaral Candidiasis.
Treasure Island: StatPearls Publishing, 2023.

73. Thomas-Ruddel DO, Schlattmann P, Pletz M, Kurzai O, Bloos F.
Risk factors for invasive candida infection in critically ill patients: A systematic review and meta-analysis.
Chest 2022;161(2):345-55.

74. Toma A, Fenaux P, Dreyfus F, Cordonnier C.
Infections in myelodysplastic syndromes.
Haematologica 2012;97(10):1459-70.

75. Urs AB, Singh H, Mohanty S, Sharma P.
Fungal osteomyelitis of maxillofacial bones: Rare presentation.
J Oral Maxillofac Pathol 2016;20(3):1-6.

76. Valdez JM, Scheinberg P, Young NS, Walsh TJ.
Infections in patients with aplastic anemia.
Semin Hematol 2009;46(3):269-76.

77. Van Grootveld R, Masarotto V, Von Dem Borne PA et al.
Effect of invasive aspergillosis on risk for different causes of death in older patients with acute myeloid leukaemia or high-risk myelodysplastic syndrome. *BMC Infect Dis 2023;23(1):1-9.*

78. Zapater E, Bagan JV, Carbonell F, Basterra J.
Malignant lymphoma of the head and neck.
Oral Dis 2010;16(2):119-128.

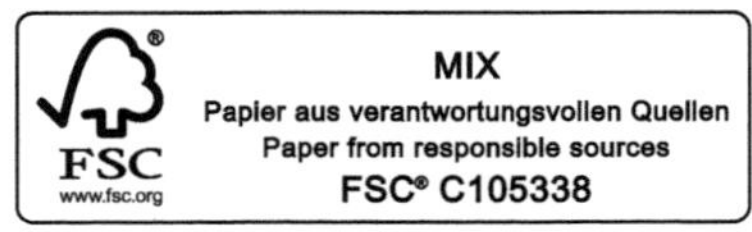

Printed by Books on Demand GmbH, Norderstedt / Germany